"Victoria Moran is the wonderful combination of dedicated yogi and gifted writer. Her words transmit the essence of compassion and calmness, with plenty of fun besides." —**Rep. Jeremy Gray**, Alabama state representative whose 2021 bill overturned a 28-year ban on teaching yoga in the state's public schools

"Victoria Moran has always spoken from the heart; her native tongue is Spirit and her teaching is truth. She has a way of weaving in history and research so that you know these things are not just her opinions, but rather holy truths to be returned to. Read and feel lifted!" —**Kathy Freston**, *New York Times* bestselling author of *Quantum Wellness*

"A feast for body and spirit, *Age Like a Yogi* draws on the time-honored teachings of both ayurveda and yoga to provide practical guidance and mystical insights for living wisely and well." —**John Robbins**, author of *Healthy at 100*

"*Age Like a Yogi* talks with you. Erudite without pedantry, transparent without that narcissistic hook, spiritual but not a hint of preach. Reading it, you feel it was written by someone who loves you." —**Loren Fishman, MD**, author of *Yoga for Osteoporosis* and *Healing Yoga*

"If you believe that life should be a meaningful adventure from start to finish, *Age Like a Yogi* is for you. Drawing on yoga's time-honored track record of promoting physical health and inner peace, this book is an honest and light-hearted companion for fully embracing every day and every decade. Highly recommended!" —**Dean Ornish, MD**, #1 *New York Times* bestselling author of *UnDo It!*

"*Age Like A Yogi* is an essential guide to living a long, vibrant and fulfilled life." —**Tara Stiles**, author of *Yoga Cures* and co-founder of Strala Yoga

"This friendly, funny, and comforting book is an invitation to enhance your vitality and experience your inner peace more fully—a winning combination at every age!" —**Meenakshi Angel Honig**, yoga instructor, wellness consultant, and author

"As a longtime yoga practitioner and woman smack dab in midlife, I'm in love with Victoria's latest book. She weaves personal anecdotes, encouraging advice, and timeless tradition into a well-rounded resource to help readers create and celebrate a dazzling third act. Prepare to be inspired—highly recommend!" —**Kimberly Wilson**, psychotherapist, author of *Advanced Tranquility*

"Victoria Moran uses yoga and ayurveda to underpin a fresh perspective on aging. With heart and actionable wisdom, *Age Like a Yogi* fills the gaps on what is often missed in our modern Western culture: a reminder that healthy aging embraces physical, mental, emotional, and spiritual components." —**Sarah Kucera, DC, CAP**, author of *The Ayurvedic Self-Care Handbook*

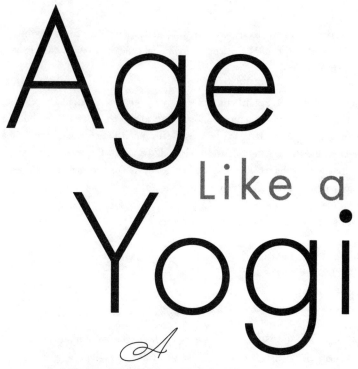

Age Like a Yogi

A HEAVENLY PATH *to a* DAZZLING THIRD ACT

VICTORIA MORAN

FOREWORD BY
SHARON GANNON

Monkfish Book Publishing Company
Rhinebeck, New York

Paperback ISBN 978-1-958972-59-5
eBook ISBN 978-1-958972-60-1

Library of Congress Cataloging-in-Publication Data

Names: Moran, Victoria, 1950- author. | Gannon, Sharon, writer of foreword.
Title: Age like a yogi : a heavenly path to a dazzling third act / Victoria
    Moran ; foreword by Sharon Gannon.
Description: Rhinebeck, New York : Monkfish Book Publishing Company, [2025]
Identifiers: LCCN 2024037374 (print) | LCCN 2024037375 (ebook) | ISBN
    9781958972595 (paperback) | ISBN 9781958972601 (ebook)
Subjects: LCSH: Yoga--Health aspects--Popular works. | Older people--Health
    and hygiene. | Aging--Physiological aspects--Popular works.
Classification: LCC RA781.7 .M658 2025 (print) | LCC RA781.7 (ebook) |
    DDC 613.7/0460846--dc23/eng/20241023
LC record available at https://lccn.loc.gov/2024037374
LC ebook record available at https://lccn.loc.gov/2024037375

Book and cover design by Colin Rolfe
Author photo from Charles Chessler Photography, NYC

Monkfish Book Publishing Company
22 East Market Street, Suite 304
Rhinebeck, New York 12572
(845) 876-4861
monkfishpublishing.com

To compassionate warriors, spiritual seekers, ageless elders,
and to Stella Cherfas who first gifted me with yoga

Contents

Foreword | Sharon Gannon   xiii

Introduction   xix

PART ONE
Age as a Spiritual Construct

1. Yoga and Extended Youthfulness   3
2. Doshas, Decades, and Your Eternal Self   7
3. Auditioning for Enlightenment   14
4. Your Bodies and Your Spirit   17

PART TWO
Moving into Maturity

5. Exercise, Physical and Metaphysical   23
6. Asana: The Proof Is in the Postures   28
7. Pranayama: A Breath of Fresh Air   35

PART THREE
Eating Peacefully

8. Yoga's Vegetarian Heritage   41
9. Today's Plant-Based Revolution   44
10. Food Over 50: Veering Toward Vata   54
11. Spices, Herbs, and Rejuvenation   58
12. Divine Dining   64

PART FOUR

Your Sacred Schedule

13. First Thing in the Morning	71
14. Each Day's Journey into Night	78
15. Seasonal Sadhana	83

PART FIVE

The Glow Factor

16. Oh, Oh, Ojas!	89
17. Happy Thoughts	93
18. Happy Chakras	96
19. Beauty Inside and Out	101
20. Skin, Hair, and Ayurveda	104

PART SIX

In Search of Sattva

21. Googling the Gunas	113
22. Get Comfy	117
23. The People Who Have Your Back	121

PART SEVEN

The Yamas: Moral Precepts

24. Ahimsa: Compassion in Action	125
25. Satya: Speak Truth, Live Truth	130
26. Asteya: There's Plenty to Go Around	133
27. Brahmacharya: Sexuality, Spirituality, Seniority	138
28. Aparigraha: Enough Already	142

PART EIGHT

Personal Disciplines

29. Saucha: Keep It Clean   147
30. Santosha: All Is Well   152
31. Tapas: Boot Camp for Yogis   156
32. Svadhyaya: Study of the Self and the Sacred   160
33. Ishvara Pranidhana: Let Go, Let God   164

PART NINE

The Soul of Yoga

34. Pratyahara: Give Your Senses a Rest   169
35. Dharana, Dhyana, Samadhi: Concentration,
    Meditation, Connection   172
36. What Kind of Yogi Are You?   177

PART TEN

Warrior Challenges

37. Dare to Live Fully   183
38. Dare to Do Your Dharma   188
39. Dare to Make Peace with Mortality   192
40. Dare to Elevate Everything   196

Brilliant Books   201
Acknowledgments and Permissions   205
About the Author   209

Foreword

When I first met Victoria Moran—it was her aura that impressed me. She radiated a childlike exuberance and enthusiasm. She was giving a public talk in a bookstore about animal rights and veganism. Her voice as well as her presence was calm, serene, and easy-going. Although the subject of her talk was very serious, there was no anger or blame infusing her message. She was confident and strong without being threatening. It was as if she was conversing with each one of us as close friends. She was communicating on a deep heart-to-heart level rather than professing—assaulting our intellects with facts to make us feel guilty. It was obvious that she cared for us and for the animals.

Because she was comfortable with herself everyone in the room felt comfortable. Her authentic smile made us want to pay attention to what she had to say, and she was beautiful in a sort of other-worldly way. I thought that she seemed so wise and well informed for someone so young. Later I learned that she was not as young as I had assumed. She reminded me of the actress and humanitarian, Audrey Hepburn, not only in her physical looks, but in her attitude about life.

When Audrey was asked in a press interview if she had any beauty tips for how to age gracefully, she replied, "For attractive lips, speak words of kindness. For lovely eyes, seek out the good in people. For a slim figure, share your food with the hungry. For beautiful hair, let a child run their fingers through it once a day. For poise, walk with the knowledge that you never walk alone. People, even more than things, have to be restored, renewed, revived, reclaimed, and redeemed; never throw anyone out of your life. Remember, if you need a helping hand, you will find one at the end of your arm. As you grow older, you will discover that you have two hands: one for helping yourself and the other for helping others."

Most everyone when they reach "a certain age," wants to look younger. We freak out when gray hairs start to sprout from our scalp and other places; we feel depressed when wrinkles and saggy skin appear. We seek out remedies to "fix" what we see as the *disease* of aging. We diet, dye our hair, apply creams, gels, masks, and lotions to our skin. We may, if we have the money, opt for cosmetic surgery or hormone replacement. We may join a gym and attempt to whip our bodies into shape. We may take a more spiritual approach and sign up for a meditation course or take up the practice of yoga. But whatever we do to make our body look and feel more youthful, it will get old and there will come a time when we want to move out of it and get a new one.

But in the meantime, what is it that we actually desire when the desire to look younger takes precedence in our life? How young do we want to look? How many years do we want to set the clock back? What age are we going for as our goal—how young is young enough?

I don't think any middle aged or 70-plus person wants to turn back the clock to look like they did when they were five years old. The youthfulness of a nubile teenager or a twenty-something is what most crave. But what is it about the look of a person at that age which is so attractive? Of course, it's the sexiness. We want to *look sexy*. Old is not considered sexy. Even the idea that an old person might be having sex creeps people out (at least young people). It seems unnatural, even perverted.

The language we use to express our thoughts has a keen impact upon our self-image. We create ourselves from the words we think and speak. To insist on dividing the world into good and bad, or young and old, is to mire ourselves in a polarity that encourages anxiety. To deem that young is good automatically says that old is bad. If young is sexy, then old must not be. All of the images that we daily download from magazines, films, and advertising condition us, kindling the desire to *look* young and to worry if we don't.

Bhava is a Sanskrit word, a yogic term, which means the ultimate good mood—a state of mind free of anxiety and other toxic negative emotions.

It is said to be our natural state of mind. Stress, anxiety, and the like are not natural to our being, but bhava is. Yogic practices are meant to help us awaken and maintain bhava—a good mood, a mood of remembrance of our soul's eternal blissful connection with God. Bhava is a mood rooted in unity—a transcendence of duality, where polarities are known but don't have an anxiety-producing effect upon our consciousness.

To begin to understand what bhava might feel like, I think the term *pronoia*, used in modern psychology to mean the opposite of paranoia, might come close. Pronoia is a state of mind where you have faith that everything will turn out for the best. You believe that the world, everyone, and every situation that you encounter is conspiring for your good. You believe that goodness will prevail over fear, anxiety, and worry, because ultimately it is goodness that is real in the eternal sense, not negativity. Goodness is an expression of truth.

From a spiritual point of view, goodness is considered real because it is eternal, and negative emotions are seen as unreal because they are temporary. Unless we are enlightened beings who have realized our eternal souls and are living liberated as *jivanmuktas*, we will identify with the relative world, who we are as a body with an ego and personality, and from time to time be seduced by negativity. We will think and identify with anger or worry, and even our words will reinforce this mistaken identity. We will declare: "I am angry, or I am afraid, or I am worried, or I am sick, or I am old and ugly." Through repetition we will convince ourselves these statements are true, and it will be more and more difficult to let them go.

These negative thoughts and emotions are experienced in your mind, but they also trigger strong physical reactions in your body—causing the release of stress hormones affecting blood pressure, heart rate, breathing and the ability to think clearly. These negative thoughts and emotions, and the stress produced by them over time, have a debilitating effect upon the cells and tissues of your body, as well as your outlook on life. They contribute to aging. To what degree a person identifies with negative thoughts and emotions, and the stress resulting from those feelings, will determine how a person ages. To put it bluntly: negative thoughts and emotions are expensive: they rob our physical cells of youthful vitality and rapidly deplete our good feelings of calm, hope, and joy.

Yoga practices provide us with ways to access our bhava, our good mood, and to let negative thoughts and emotions go. The practices offer us ways to transcend time, freeing us from the haunting memories of our past and worry about our future. Such thoughts trigger stress, and stress causes aging.

Yoga philosophy puts emphasis on the *atha*, which translates from Sanskrit into the present moment, the now. The present moment contains infinite possibilities; it is the only reality that actually exists. The past is gone and the future nonexistent. Through yogic practices like the *yamas* and *niyamas* (ethical guidelines), *asana* (relationship to the Earth), *pranayama* (conscious breathing), meditation, prayer, and *mantra* (recitation of God's names), a person can let go of worrying about the past and the future and enter into the present. When these practices are engaged in regularly, meaning when they become part of a person's daily life, one is able to live in the present. The more a person chooses to live in the present and embrace the creative potential that the present offers, the more aware they will become of their eternal, luminous soul. A person like this will be less likely to be seduced by anxieties produced by ego and caught up in the net of negativity.

The Yoga Sutras of Patanjali describe a person who is able to live in the present, free from anxieties about the past and the future. He introduces an interesting idea about such a person when he says: If a person can let go of tendencies toward greediness and become more selfless and generous, not taking more than they need, then they will experience the present moment; and they will come to know their destiny—the creative purpose of their life will be realized. For example, *aparigraha*, a Sanskrit term in the Yoga Sutras and throughout Eastern thought, means greedlessness.

APARIGRAHA-STHAIRYE JANMA-KATHANTA-SAMBODHAH (II.39)

People don't grow old. When they stop growing, they become old. Swami Satchidananda said, "Yoga teachings provide a path to an easeful body, a peaceful mind, and a useful life. If you are becoming more ease-ful, peaceful, and useful, then you know you are growing." The definition of an adult is someone who has stopped growing. Let us resist this idea of adulthood and cultivate a childlike optimism—a ready belief in the goodness of life. Reality is our perception of it. We see the reflection in the mirror and judge it according to how we see it.

The good news is that we can shift our perception of reality. What we perceive as reality is only limited by our imagination. Imagination is governed by creativity. Nothing in this material world is stable; every-thing and everyone is subject to time and thus change. How we expe-rience reality is determined by how creative we allow ourselves to be. Children, artists, and yogis experience the warping of time that occurs in the midst of creative endeavor. When children are deep into playing, the hands of the clock seem to stop moving. Something similar happens to artists who become lost in a creative project. Yogis in meditation report that they enter into a realm where time seems to be suspended. Could there be a connection between creativity and youthfulness?

This book explores the subject of aging from a yogic perceptive. Victoria sites Patanjali's yoga sutra, an ancient self-help book, and shares with us some of the wisdom contained that has provided her with valuable insights into the quest for youthful aging. Sexiness does have something to do with it. Sex and creativity are linked. According to the yoga sutras, the energy associated with the second chakra is creative energy and includes sexual energy. The Yoga Sutras say that when a person does not misuse this sexual creative energy, they will be endowed with vitality, good health, and youthful energy. Some commentators go so far as to describe the effects of *brahmach-arya* as palatable charisma—an irresistible magnetism. Such a person can light up a room, as was evident to me when I met Victoria Moran.

BRAHMACHARYA-PRATISTHAYAM VIRYA-LABHAH (II.38)

Brahmacharya is spoken about in the Yoga Sutras, in the "ethical guide-lines" section. It is a practice where a person respects the creative power, which includes the power of sex, and does not abuse it by manipulating others. Every animal raised on a farm to be turned into meat and eaten is sexually abused; knowing this fact provides enough incentive for me to be vegan, maybe for you too?

Every living person, human as well as all animals (and maybe even trees), has an eternal soul that animates the person from an inner luminosity glowing with divine light. That inner light is creative energy, and it can be suppressed or nurtured by the actions we take and the thoughts and emotions we choose to identify with. When that light is nurtured, it expands and can be felt by others around you. The glow that emanates from a creative, kind, and caring person is warm and enveloping, whereas selfish people tend to be dim and contracted, stifling their soul's inner light, and we don't feel welcome in their presence. A yogi's body glows with warmth radiating from within, expanding outward into their aura.

SAMANA-JAYAJ JVALANAM (III.41)

Yoga practice is designed to free us from the tyranny of the selfish ego and allow us to realize that who we really are is a joyful, immortal soul encased in a body—a body that will eventually die. With that knowledge we can turn our attention to how best to live. We all die according to how we have lived, so the best way to prepare for a good death is to live a good life. No matter how long we live, life will be brief. Before you know it, your life will be over, and it will be time to die—again. In the epic Hindu poem, the Mahabharata, King Yudhishthira is asked, "Of all things in life, what is the most amazing?" He answers, "That a person, seeing others die all around them, never thinks that they will die." The fact that you are alive and here now is something to gratefully celebrate. Life provides us with opportunities to learn through love, kindness, and forgiveness. Yoga provides us with practical wisdom, to help us awaken to the knowledge of who we really are—luminous ageless souls.

Sharon Gannon is a yoga teacher, animal rights advocate, musician, author, dancer, and choreographer. Along with David Life, she is co-founder of the Jivamukti Yoga method.

Introduction

In my early twenties, I worked as a library admin at the Illinois head-quarters of the Theosophical Society in America. Theosophy is Eastern philosophy packaged for Western consumption in the late 1800s by spiritual adventurers who had journeyed to India and Tibet. They returned with zeitgeist-shifting accounts of enlightened teachers living in the Himalayas, and with a staunch commitment to the essential oneness of all people and all beings. When we needed an extra hand in the library, we'd call on Iris, a stunning septuagenarian who lived locally and whose study of eclectic spirituality had spanned decades. The braids neatly wrapped around her head were glistening white like cotton snow at Christmastime, the kind with the glittery pieces; and when she smiled, she momentarily became the shining star at the top of the tree.

It didn't matter if the problem was pilfered books, a backlog of unanswered messages, or the fallout of a lecture the night before, with volumes on mysticism, personal development, and the world's religions misshelved or left in careless piles on tables and chairs and the grand piano. Iris regarded it all as delight in the making. Once when I was complaining about some aggravation or other, she lit up in that way she had and responded, "The darling physical plane!" This probably makes sense only if you already see physical reality as a yogi would, as one "plane" of many and far from the most appealing. I knew only that despite supposedly having the bloom of youth on my side, Iris had the glow and I did not.

A preternaturally serious young person, I wondered if Iris's incessant positivity might belie some variant of Alzheimer's. Perhaps she'd simply forgotten that the world was a mess. As I came to know her better, though, and as more people like her came into my life, the pathology hypothesis couldn't hold up. I was the one with dementia: I had failed to remember who I was.

I've spent much of the half-century since—when I wasn't distracted by wanting to lose weight, or be loved back, or have Oprah know my name—attempting to remember. In this quest, I earned a degree in comparative religions, traveled to India and Tibet like those old-time theosophists, and visited—each time with the sincere intention of remaining—so many philosophies and spiritual systems that I came to chime in with theologian Marcus Bach who called himself a "vagabond in the wonderful world of spirit."

What has kept me grounded through all the searching and seeking is yoga, there at the center of things since I discovered it at 17. At that time, in my part of the world anyway, yoga was largely a misunderstood oddity, to be filed away under "foreign, probably dangerous." For me that made it even more captivating. There were three books on the subject in the downtown library in Kansas City, Missouri, my hometown. Two of them had to do with aging: *Forever Young, Forever Healthy*, by Indra Devi, an intrepid Russian woman instrumental in disseminating yoga to twenti-eth-century America, and *Yoga, Youth, and Reincarnation*, by journalist Jess Stern. I was certain I'd never be old, but that didn't keep me from checking out the books repeatedly and reading them time and again.

The following year I moved to London to study fashion, but found myself far more intrigued by inner explorations, participating in silent worship at the Friends Meeting House just north of Trafalgar Square and discovering nearby a magical shop called Watkins, specializing in books about spirituality. That's where I learned of my first yoga teacher, Stella Cherfas. She is ninety-eight now, still teaches a chair yoga class once a week, and lives in a second-floor walkup—that's third floor in American. Stella is a role model who encourages me to proceed with courage and humor, as well as meditation, deep breathing, and dark chocolate in the morning.

As echoed in the Perennial Philosophy of Aldous Huxley and others, yoga states that at the core of every genuine spiritual teaching is a mystical nucleus which connects it with every other genuine spiritual teaching. In addition, every living entity is an expression of universal consciousness which "resides in the middle of the body," according to the Katha Upanishad. In a somewhat more metaphorical vein, transcendentalist Ralph Waldo Emerson wrote, "Every man is a divinity is disguise, a god playing the fool." And Rumi, a Sufi, poeticized, "I looked in churches, temples, and mosques, but I found the Divine within my heart."

Getting in touch with this part that's way cooler than our regular self but is, in fact, our true Self, is the foundation of yoga—and of aging yogically. It gives us what we need in the moment: beauty, consolation, courage, or an idea so bright we have to look around to be sure it didn't come from somebody who's read more books or has more credentials. The tools you'll need are collected here for you. Some deal with the body, others with the soul, and you won't be too far in before you realize that what you do for one benefits the other.

Yoga is far more a practice than a belief system, although there are beliefs shared by most serious adherents. These are components of a worldview formulated thousands of years ago in India by sages called *rishis* who, somewhat like the Hebrew prophets of the Bible, had direct revelation of universal truths. One of the most inviting parts of this philosophy is that it regards all positive paths of meaning-making as valid. The Rig Veda, a text dated from 1500 to 1000 BCE, states, "Truth is one. Sages call it by various names."

Therefore, even though yogic teachings share some tenets and terminology with the Hindu religion that developed at the same time and place, yoga is not a religion and can be practiced by anyone of any religion or none. When I was starting out and wanted to be sure I wasn't going to be at odds with the faith in which I grew up, I read a reassuring book called *Christian Yoga* by a French Benedictine priest, Father Jean-Marie Déchanet. Today, there is even a nonprofit organization called Christians Practicing Yoga "that values and honors the intersection of yoga philosophy and Christian theology" (www.christianspracticingyoga.com).

Whatever your belief system, you might bump into yogic concepts that contradict it or appear to. Reincarnation is one example. This has always seemed plausible to me: even as a toddler I felt certain I'd been somewhere before this. Yoga accepts without question that we are travelers, inhabiting many physical forms the way one might stay at a string of hotels, B&Bs, and campgrounds on a cross-country road trip. Of course, not everybody shares this view. My own husband is one of them. When I met William, his sole interest in anything spiritual was a fondness for *Jesus Christ Superstar*, but in his sixties, he went to seminary and was ordained as an Interfaith minister. These days, we have rich conversations around faith and purpose and the meaning of life, but we remain on opposite sides of the reincarnation question. He's a one-and-done person. If you are, too, no worries. Yoga is a buffet, not a set menu.

In my life, aging like a yogi incorporates what I've learned studying spiritual systems with their roots in India (including yoga, Vedanta, theosophy—clearly different for scholars, but for me an expansive, interrelated teaching), as well as Christian and Jewish mysticism, the 12-Step programs, and New Thought, the late nineteenth-century American movement that brought to the fore such concepts as positive thinking and the interconnectedness of body, mind, and spirit. If something suggested in this book doesn't resonate with you, move on to the next idea. Back burners are ideal places for slow-simmered stews and for notions that could—maybe someday, maybe not—turn out to be delicious.

Out of respect for yoga tradition, I will provide the names that these concepts were given in the original Sanskrit. The English follows immediately, though, so you'll never find yourself lost in translation. When it comes to yoga asanas or postures, however, I will generally stick with English. These terms are now in the vernacular of Western gym culture, so let's keep things simple. In addition, we'll stay with the practically applicable aspects of teachings that can go very deep indeed.

The purpose of this book is not necessarily to turn you into a "yoga person" unless you already are one, or yoga captures your imagination so thoroughly that you want to immerse yourself in it. It is, rather, to familiarize you with the grammar of yoga so you can start right away to apply select elements to rejuvenate your body and uplift your life. For example, you don't have to do formal breath control exercises to breathe a little more deeply and consciously on your walk tomorrow morning.

Many of the tips I offer about the care of our physical selves come from yoga's sister science, *ayurveda*, which means "knowledge of life." These two bodies of wisdom grew up alongside each other. Despite the prevailing contemporary view that yoga is only a way to exercise, an alternative to Pilates or barre classes, it was, and is, primarily about spiritual growth. Its well-known postures came into being fairly late in its history as a means to develop a body that would harmoniously house an evolving spirit.

Ayurveda, while spiritually inspired, is about physical wellness and is recognized today by the World Health Organization as a viable health-care system. It is as detailed as Western medicine, with branches including internal medicine, pediatrics, surgery, and more. While ayurveda was forced underground when India was a British colony, there are now eight million ayurvedic *vaidyas* (doctors) on the subcontinent, and over 3,000 ayurvedic hospitals. Even so, *Age Like a Yogi* is not a medical text and I am not a doctor, ayurvedic or otherwise. Contained within ayurveda, however, is a rich do-it-yourself component for life enhancement and self-care. This is where we'll focus.

I also share ayurveda as I understand it and as it has benefitted me. I have tremendous respect for the system, but I don't blindly follow every precept. For example, traditional ayurvedic teachings revere dairy, particularly ghee (clarified butter). I am a committed vegan. That's okay. It is ardently yogic that the Inner Teacher gets the final say.

And just as I am not a physician, I'm not Indian, not in this life anyway. At the present time, the accusation of cultural appropriation is often brought against anyone who shares wisdom that has a birthplace other than their own. As you already know, I come from the American Midwest, and that's where yoga found me as a curious teenager looking for God in the public library.

I believe that these teachings were first a gift from the Infinite and then a gift from India to anyone on earth who is open to receive them gratefully and reverently. The teachers who brought them from India to America and beyond—pioneers such as Swami Vivekananda in 1893 (The Vedanta Society), Paramahansa Yogananda in 1920 (Self-Realization Fellowship), Swami Prabhupada in 1966 (International Society of Krishna Consciousness)—would surely have saved themselves the trip had they not intended for us to learn from them and season the broth of yoga with some flavorings of our own.

For me, these flavorings come not only from various spiritual teachings but from the Irises I've known, spiritual teachers and friends who could pass for sages any day of the week. Many of these have been women of a certain age. Although we'd be hard-pressed to find a group in society more dismissed than "little old ladies," women in their later years are unparalleled repositories of spiritual wealth. We live in a culture that pressures us to hide "telltale signs of aging" and cautions us to avoid revealing the number of times we have, in one remarkable body, circumnavigated the sun. It is those trips, however, that christened our teachers *wise women* and that are in the process of doing the same for us.

This is to dismiss neither spiritual wunderkind, old souls in young bodies who offer bright, fresh takes on timeworn tenets, nor men and other gender-identified people. Their wisdom will show up here, too, along with some insights that have come to me from within, from the still small voice I finally accepted as real after repeatedly ignoring it at my peril. And your voice from inside is your lodestar—not the wishful thinking that can masquerade as your inner voice, nor the internal critic that provokes you to second-guess yourself, but that calm, deep sense of "Oh, yeah—this is the real deal."

My hope is that you'll find here ideas that resonate with your own and practices that make you feel happier and more alive. If I get my way, what you'll read will nestle nicely alongside the spiritual life you already have, whether you think you don't have one yet or you haven't missed morning meditation in twenty-five years. And just so you know, I will be thinking of you going forward, that you'll spend a lot of time amazed and almost none afraid. That's when you'll discover that aging like a yogi is nothing other than growing into yourself—and that all your inner light ever needed to shine like the dickens was for you to know that it was there.

Part One

....

Age as a Spiritual Construct

Chapter 1

Yoga and Extended Youthfulness

*You can free yourself from aging by reinterpreting your
body and by grasping the link between belief and biology.*

....

DEEPAK CHOPRA, MD

The first high school reunion I attended was not my own, but I knew
that the strangers I was meeting had birthdates within a year of one
another. Astoundingly, some of the grads looked as if they were still in
high school, while a few could have passed for their grandparents. That
was the first time it struck me how differently people age—and I was
looking only at the outside, the part that matters least.

Even then, in my mid-twenties, I'd been around yoga long enough
to know, intellectually anyhow, that while we *live* in mortal bodies, we
are immortal spirit. Not only that: the same yogic lifestyle that nurtures
and develops the soul also impacts the body and the rate at which it ages.
But in that hotel banquet hall, with its white tablecloths and popular
open bar, the theoretical became practical: *Each of us has the choice to age
randomly, taking our chances with genetic roulette, or we can age like a yogi.*

Modern medicine calls the postponement of pathology in later life
"mitigation of morbidity." This means that if you live to be ninety, you
get to be fully alive for ninety years, or eighty-nine and some months,
instead of spending twenty years or more embroiled in discomfort and
decline. Yoga and its sister science, ayurveda, have been mitigating morbidity for several thousand years.

Aging well draws on a combination of factors. These include our hereditary mapping, past exposure to toxic chemicals or excess sunlight, physical accidents and emotional traumas, and the eating, drinking, sleeping, moving, working, and thinking norms throughout our lives. In addition to genetics and lifestyle, culture influences how people age. Dan Buettner's seminal book, *The Blue Zones*, which looked at places around the globe where people were living both long and well, showed that in societies where elders are revered, where everyone has a role in community life and where being active and productive in one's eighties and nineties is expected, robust longevity is common.

Western urban and suburban mores tend to be the opposite of this, but we can create personal blue zones using tools from yoga and ayurveda. These systems are life-altering, sacred even, and the wisdom that resides within you is a super-system. When yoga does what it's meant to, it connects you to this wisdom, starting with an acknowledgment of who you really are.

We don't get into metaphysical verities in our daily transactions, nor do we need to. If you ask who I am, I'll say, "Victoria Moran." Okay, but that's a married name; I used to have a different one. "I'm in my seventies." True, but I was once seventeen and may one day be eighty-seven. "I live in New York City." Well, I have for twenty-five years. I didn't start out here, though, and I have no way of knowing where I'll end up. While my answers are not inaccurate, they do prompt the question: If everything in my elevator speech is conditional, who am I really? And who are you?

According to the sages, we are divine and eternal, embodied now as individuals with the task of remembering the divine and eternal part. In order to age like a yogi, you do not have to become a Sanskrit scholar or a philosophy major, but you will run into the terms that follow, so I want to introduce them. Don't worry about learning them. Anything you need for your personal journey will naturally stick.

- *Brahman* is the Sanskrit word for the formless, unknowable Absolute; think Source, First Cause, Alpha and Omega, the Force from *Star Wars*.

- *Atman*, spirit, is that same divine essence but alive within us: boundless, timeless, and perfect. Atman is sometimes described as Self—that capital S differentiates this Self from our ego or personality. For me, Atman is what George Fox, founder of the Quakers (Society of Friends), referred to as "that of God in every man."

- *Jiva* translates as "soul" and reflects Atman. It is universal consciousness individualized, appearing as finite and separate so we can experience our lives as unique entities.

The upshot is that we are not simply created by God, we are expressions of God, or whatever concept of great Love and Power works for you. (And that Power is the awe-inspiring, cosmic kind, not military-industrial complex stuff.)

These concepts are not limited to Indian thought. I remember a nun in third grade catechism class explaining how God made us from himself, because there was nothing else. If you're more comfortable with the familiar, just think of your inner being as soul or spirit or whatever word you like. Terminology aside, that inner being is the real you, and it does not age. The more thoroughly you can identify with the part of yourself that has been you all your life, the more youthful you will feel and appear.

Do you remember Iris in the library? (She was in the Introduction.) Iris was a beauty as she approached 80 because she had been relating to her inner being for so long that she remained young in all the ways that mattered. She was not immune from every indicator of the passage of time—her hair was white and there were lines on her face, especially when she laughed, which she did often—but everything about the way she came across expressed vitality and a youthful sense of wonder. This can happen for anyone who chooses to age like a yogi.

PRACTICES FOR THE PATH

Before your feet touch the floor in the morning, entertain the concept that you are not your body or your mind and certainly not the age on your driver's license. The yogis would say that you are the eternal Atman and that affirming this often is a good idea. If that's not a concept that resonates with you, use one that does, such as, "I am a divine creation" or "I matter to the universe."

Chapter 2

Doshas, Decades, and Your Eternal Self

*If your body and mind were a hand-written story, then
vata is the ink, pitta is the pen, and kapha is the paper.
Each one is vital.*

....

KAITLIN LACEY, RYT-500

According to the teachings of both yoga and ayurveda, the fundamental cause of illness is forgetting who we are: immortal Spirit,
Atman or Self, now inhabiting a physical body. Because the Self doesn't
age, the less than welcome aspects of later life are delayed when we identify more with that eternal essence than with our physical being which
has an expiration date, even for those of us who get our checkups and
eat our vegetables.

At the very outset of the Yoga Sutras of Patanjali, the second century BCE text that codified *raja yoga*, the royal path of yoga we are
exploring here, we read *"yogas citta vritti nirodhah,"* the classic line that
translates as "Yoga is the restraint of the fluctuations of the mind." Full
stop. Everything else we know as yoga operates in support of this goal,
because those fluctuations distract us from recognizing our true nature.

Nevertheless, we're housed in a body. We filter all impressions
through a brain. We express ourselves through personalities. Enter
ayurveda. This sibling system is concerned with our manifest selves and
dovetails with yoga to provide us with the best possible lives. Ayurveda
is elemental—literally. The basic elements of the physical world—earth,
air, ether (space), fire, and water—also make up our physical bodies, the

focus of ayurveda. We can think of the aim of yoga as perfect peace and the aim of ayurveda, perfect health.

As *sister* sciences, not cloned ones, they sometimes make contradictory suggestions. For example, ayurveda favors cooked food—not all cooked all the time, but most of the time for most people. This is because cooked food is believed to be easier to digest than salads and smoothies. The warmth is nurturing in cold and damp seasons, and our systems don't have to do the work to heat the food to body temperature. Yoga, on the other hand, looks at all the activities of daily life, including how we eat, as opportunities to help refine our bodies and free our spirit. Therefore, yogis tend to favor light fare, with plenty of fresh fruits and vegetables just as they come from nature. Indicative of this was the announcement of famous twentieth-century guru, Satya Sai Baba, that the ideal foods for humans are ripe banana and young coconut.

So, what are we to do, we regular people who want to live well, age well, *and* mature into spiritually aware human beings? It lies somewhere in the middle. Isn't that almost always the case? You listen to your intuition, use your good sense, mix the best of modern science with the most resonant ancient wisdom, and find your way. Ayurveda helps you find your particular way by defining and describing your unique psycho-physical self, your *prakriti* or constitution.

THREE ENERGIES CALLED DOSHAS

This combination of energies depicting the five elements is solidified at the moment of conception as your body type. It is a composite of three energies called *doshas*. Their names are *vata*, *pitta*, and *kapha*. Everybody has all three, but one usually dominates, either being markedly more prominent than the other two, or somewhat more prominent than the runner-up dosha.

The pattern codified for you is for life and, like Baby Bear's porridge, it is just right. What happens, however, is that stress comes on the scene via food that isn't right for us, too little sleep (or sleeping at the wrong hours), too much work, too little exercise, temperature extremes, and emotional upheavals. These cause one or more of the doshas to increase within us, leading to imbalance, the precursor of disease.

While learning your body type is always interesting, it sometimes solves mysteries that are decades old. *Why do I get anxiety in situations that make other people angry? Why am I prone to skin breakouts? Why can I never lose the ten pounds that bother me, even though I know for a fact that I eat less than a lot of other people?* Knowing about the doshas can also be a boon to relationships, as when you realize, for example, that the spouse who likes to crank up the heat in winter isn't trying to make you hot and sweaty. They are cold and can't understand why you're not.

To get a serious read on your prakriti, your basic doshic makeup, and your *vikruti*, the imbalances you may be dealing with now, it is ideal to see a trained ayurvedic practitioner. After an in-depth questionnaire and interview, the practitioner will examine your pulses (in ayurveda, pulse diagnosis is an in-depth study, far more complex than "taking a pulse"), your tongue, your eyes, and your fingernails, allowing your body itself to reveal its doshic blueprint. Lacking this, you can take a dosha quiz. I like Dr. Deepak Chopra's (www.deepakchopra.com/doshaquiz) and the one on the Banyan Botanicals website (www.banyanbotanicals.com/doshaquiz). Banyan Botanicals is an ayurvedic store that's also a rich source of information on ayurveda; making a purchase is not necessary to take the quiz. When you answer the questions, don't overthink. The first response that comes to mind is best.

Any good dosha quiz asks the same questions more than once in different ways. That's intentional. It may ask, for example, if your skin is dry or oily. It may have been oily earlier in your life but dry now, so you may be confounded as to how to answer. Just put down the first response that comes to mind. It will probably ask in another section if your hair is dry or oily and that answer, in concert with the one about your skin and all the other questions, will help provide the total picture.

You are not looking to "balance out" your doshas and have one-third of each. A small percentage of folks are like that. They're called *tri-doshic*. That's fine, but they are no better—and no healthier—than anybody else. Your doshic formula, the one you were born with, is perfect.

If you're 80 percent pitta, 15 percent kapha, and 5 percent vata, that's terrific. If you're 60 percent vata, 30 percent pitta, and 10 percent kapha, excellent. This is really encouraging after decades of hearing what was wrong with us. "Your weight is supposed to be this much, and your measurements these, and your athletic abilities better than they are." Thank goodness some of this should-i-ness has dissolved from Western culture, and there's more room to be different in the twenty-first century than there was in the twentieth. Ayurveda, to its credit, has celebrated diversity from its beginnings.

Our challenge, then, is not to make ourselves over but to stay as close as possible to our original doshic makeup throughout our lives. This can be tricky because the time of the day, the season of the year, and the stages of a life are all influenced by a particular dosha. Such realities as a late night, an incompatible meal, or an upsetting confrontation, even when unavoidable, affect the doshas too. When you find yourself with too much of any one of them, emotional or physical troubles can result. For that person we described as 80 percent pitta, too much might be 85 percent. For our second hypothetical person, the one whose natural makeup is 30 percent pitta, having that go up to 35 or 40 percent could be too much.

We will explore later where imbalances come from, but to give you a general idea of the doshas themselves, let's start from the ground up with the earthiest among them.

Kapha

Kapha elements are earth and water, so there is a heaviness to this dosha, a steadiness, a reliability. Regardless of our individual prakriti, all of us are strongly influenced by kapha dosha in childhood. Kapha bodies are a bit round and fleshy by nature, although kapha people lack the voracious appetite of an unbalanced pitta or the tendency to snack mindlessly as a vata might when trying to feel grounded. Kapha is a connoisseur of comfort and will get it whenever possible. Therefore, this person would do well to go for a weekend hike or bike ride, while jittery vata or pissed-off pitta might do well with a spa day or meditation retreat.

Since it can be hard for kapha to get moving, ayurveda eases its general discouragement of caffeine and allows coffee for kaphas; they can use the boost. Because kapha energy moves slowly, people in whom it predominates are slow to become ill, although an out-of-balance kapha person can be prone to respiratory infections, with or without lung involvement, and to obesity-related disorders. Kept in balance with light, high-fiber foods (think warming whole grains paired with fresh vegetables and spices) and regular exercise, kapha is apt to remain healthy—and generous, kind, attractive, and good-natured—well into old age. Some kaphas we recognize are Deepak Chopra, Martin Luther King, Jr., Oprah Winfrey, and Jennifer Lopez.

Pitta

Pitta (fire and water) folks are apt to be mid-sized, muscular, and the ones in the room asking if someone can open a window. In balance, they're quick, strategic thinkers, strong and dependable, with unparalleled executive ability. Many of the people heading organizations, commanding troops, or commanding attention as public speakers are pitta dominant. Pitta is most active in all of us from about sixteen to fifty-five, when its drive and ambition help us establish a career, raise a family, look out for aging parents, and secure our future.

Out of balance, a pitta person can be angry, rude, and opinionated, and develop inflammatory conditions ranging from skin rashes to acid reflex and ulcers. Since pitta is hot and excitable by nature, a spicy Mexican meal with a few shots of tequila isn't a great choice for them. Even though ayurveda discourages iced drinks and frosty treats (these douse *agni*, the digestive fire), a pitta person is least impacted by this indulgence. Pittas stay happy when the purpose they crave and the passion they are filled with are balanced by ample rest, regular meals, and an abundance of sweet, juicy fruits—melons, figs, oranges, mangos. Pittas to picture: John F. Kennedy, Serena Williams, Jennifer Aniston.

Vata

Vata is called the "king of the doshas" because it governs movement and all biological activity, and vata-dominant people tend to be active. Vata's elements, air and ether, give high-vata types a light build and sensitivity to cold and wind. When they are in balance, creative, curious vata peeps have a lovely light-heartedness that enables them to lift a stale or somber mood. When out of balance, they're likely to feel restless or exhausted but unable to sleep soundly; they may experience digestive disorders or osteoarthritis symptoms.

Caffeine can put anxious vata types over the edge. And an iced coffee for this cold dosha pushes them even further out of balance. Ditto carbonated beverages: vata is aerated by nature. On the other hand, steamy ginger or licorice tea, or spiced almond milk (in ayurveda, blanched almonds are a specific for vata) would be comforting. Keeping warm and hydrated, staying out of drafts, and avoiding upsetting or violent images are good tips for vata, as is sticking to a steady schedule and allowing ample time to recover from travel and time zone changes. At mealtimes, warm, soothing, easily digestible foods are all balancing for this dosha (details in chapter 10). Iconic vatas: Audrey Hepburn, Fred Astaire, Barack Obama.

Vata dosha tends to exert itself after menopause (andropause for men), and become more pronounced as years pass. The basic template for our individual constitution remains, but few of us make it to sixty without seeing signs of increasing vata. Some of these can be positive. For example, if we've long expressed the quick-to-anger, everything-is-an-emergency aspects of out-of-balance pitta, we might find ourselves in later life with more patience and understanding, helping keep us in that enviable category of elders whose blood pressure stays right on target.

On the other hand, the encroachment of vata makes for dryer skin and hair. We might start to see the bones and veins in our hands. The roundness leaves our faces and some opt for fillers from the dermatologist. We seem to need a sweater when other people don't. Foods we used to digest with ease may cause gas or constipation. We might notice for the first time some stiffness or creakiness in our joints.

All this—any of it, really—could lead to distress about getting old. While a great gift of yoga is acceptance of life as it is, getting old included, we can calm vata dosha and lessen its influence on our body and emotions. We will learn in some of the upcoming chapters more ways to work with vata to make living in a vintage body nearly as comfortable as living in one right off the showroom floor. A simple, effective formula for aging well is this: *Pacify vata for a calm, well-functioning mind and body, and allow yoga to remind you daily that the true Self is beyond both mind and body.*

PRACTICES FOR THE PATH

Take a dosha quiz, and then treat yourself to a dosha-discovery gift. Any little self-care indulgence works, but let me recommend a spice blend, called a churna, specifically formulated for your prominent dosha. (You might also order Vata Churna to help calm the dosha that creeps up on all of us in maturity.) One source for these special blends is Maharishi Ayurvedic Products, www.mapi.com.

Chapter 3

Auditioning for Enlightenment

Jesus recognized that God within him and became Christ.
So did Siddhartha Gautama
and became Buddha. So did I. And so can you.

....

ABHIJIT NASKAR, *NEURONS OF JESUS*

K nowing your dosha type so you can work to support your unique physical presentation is one common-sense step to take for living well now and in the future. But there's a bigger picture. Yoga starts healing your life the moment you understand that our time on earth is, fundamentally, an audition for enlightenment. Of course, we are also here to learn, share our talents, experience joy, ease suffering, right wrongs, and have loving and supportive relationships with others. But all these are in addition to and in support of the momentous process of Self-realization.

This idea also shows up in Western theology and philosophy. Pierre Teilhard de Chardin, paleontologist and Catholic priest, spoke of the soul's evolution as a journey from unconscious perfection to conscious imperfection to conscious perfection. It is a long trip. That's why yogis (and some priests, if not in public) espouse reincarnation. Either way, all that matters for your life to have an astonishing amount of meaning is to own that everything you're engaged in and everything you're going through is an opportunity to discover who you are. Like, who you *really* are.

Every time of life is optimal for something. We know that early childhood is ideal for learning languages. Experts say that the late twenties and early thirties (30.5 to be exact) is the peak time for giving birth. And later life—after fifty, or sixty, or seventy—is the perfect time to get to know your Self, your inner light, God even, if you're okay with that word.

If you ask a hundred people to name the most spiritual person they have ever known, I'll bet fifty will say "my grandmother." This is because Nana took the time to develop her soul. Surely, we can access the Great Beneficence at any age, but early on God has a lot of competition for our time and energy. We are living in this impressive world in a flashy new body. There's so much to discover and experience. Then sex shows up and demands attention. Family and career ask a lot. We might devote decades to making our mark or to working hard just to get by. In either case, it's often not until later life that many of us get around to seeing that all we've done for all this time, and what lies ahead, is really about our soul making its way back home.

In traditional Hindu culture, in which auditioning for enlightenment is a given, life is divided into four stages:

- *Brahmacharya*, our time as a student, when we both learn how to navigate the material world and are introduced to moral and religious teachings. (This same word, used differently, is one of the precepts of yoga.)
- *Grihastha*, the householder period when we establish a home, family, career, reputation. Deepak Chopra calls this the fame-and-fortune phase.
- *Vanaprastha*, traditionally the state of the hermit or forest dweller; in modern times, it is retirement, with the opportunity to perform more *seva*, service, through volunteering or a second career devoted to the well-being of others, and taking more time for spiritual study and inner work.
- *Sannyasa*, traditionally the time of renunciation, turning from the world to devote oneself entirely to spiritual practice and discovery. (A few people, such as cloistered monks and nuns, spend their whole lives in the sannyasa phase.)

Spiritual seekers embody these stages in the West, as well. When I lived at Theosophical Society headquarters in my early twenties, I was one of a handful of idealistic young people in a houseful of retirees, giving the experience they had gleaned in the business world to the running of the Society. Many of them did this vanaprastha work into their late sixties and seventies and then went on to a second retirement (sannyasa), when the pull of the inner quest was stronger even than that of outward service.

It is a grace to know about these stages and the value of each one. When advancing age seems hellbent on making us smaller, we can look within, where things have never been better. Life illuminates when you understand that any task can be spiritual practice. Getting that medical test or filling out forms for Social Security is no longer a dreary chore to postpone. It's audition material.

I invite you to determine an approximation of where you are within the four life stages, and take a moment to be in awe of the promise of the place at which you find yourself. There is likely to be some overlap. Maybe you've retired from your job but you still have a child at home, and you're in graduate school to prepare for work in a humanitarian endeavor that may or not be paid. This scenario has the householder and student stages superimposed on the retirement phase. It's all right on time doin' fine. Just be aware that, even amidst modern busyness, the inner life matters, and it will matter more as you go along. Make room for meditation, contemplation, spiritual study, and time spent in nature and with other people who are consciously on a spiritual path. You're up for a really big role. Prioritize the audition.

PRACTICES FOR THE PATH

Choose a day this week when you will consciously audition for enlightenment all day long. If you observe a sabbath, use that day. Otherwise, just pick one: Meaningful Monday, Wisdom Wednesday, Sanctified Saturday. On this day, put your spiritual life front and center. Focus on service, generosity, meditation, spreading joy, and blessing everybody from the neighbor you visit to the bulbs you plant. If this proves fulfilling, maybe you'll do Meaningful Monday (or whatever day you choose) every week.

Chapter 4

Your Bodies and Your Spirit

*Understanding ourselves through the five koshas provides
a 360-degree view of what it means to be fully human
and deeply self-aware. Then we can consciously choose to
make changes ... or find ... peace of mind
if change is not possible*

....

BETH GIBBS, AUTHOR OF *ENLIGHTEN UP!*

Bodies plural? Yes, we have a whole constellation of them. If you have trouble wrapping your mind around this notion, it can help to remember that we often allude to our physical being in metaphorical ways. For example:

- "She hurt my feelings." *I'm sorry that happened. Where are the feelings she hurt?*
- "I love him with all my heart." *Beautiful. Does that mean your heart flutters? Speeds up? Misses a beat?*
- "I should have listened to my gut." *It always seems to be right, doesn't it? But was it a burning esophagus, a queasy tummy, a bowel acting irritable?*

Yoga would say that these sensations, which may have little or nothing to do with our standard senses, are seated in one of our "subtle" bodies, layers of being. Called *koshas* in Sanskrit, all our bodies—physical, etheric, mental, astral, and bliss—reside within one another the way a sword fits in its sheath, and "sheath" is the literal meaning of kosha. In the box, you will see how these are described in the original text; I've added the Sanskrit names parenthetically.

THE FIVE BODIES, TAITTIRIYA UPANISHAD, SIXTH CENTURY BCE

Human beings consist of a material body (*annamaya kosha*) built from the food they eat. Those who care for this body are nourished by the universe itself.

Inside this is another body made of life energy (*pranamaya kosha*). It fills the physical body and takes its shape. Those who treat this vital force as divine, experience excellent health and longevity because this energy is the source of physical life.

Within the vital force is yet another body, this one made of thought energy (*manomaya kosha*). It fills the two denser bodies and has the same shape. Those who understand and control the mental body are no longer afflicted by fear.

Deeper still lies another body comprised of intellect (*vijnanamaya kosha*). It permeates the three denser bodies and assumes the same form. Those who establish their awareness here free themselves from unhealthy thoughts and actions, and develop the self-control necessary to achieve their goals.

Hidden inside it is yet a subtler body, composed of pure joy (*anandamaya kosha*). It pervades the other bodies and shares the same shape. It is experienced as happiness, delight, and bliss.

These bodies, nesting within you like Russian dolls, are energetic layers wrapping up your precious essence. Lucky for us, self-care applies to all parts of ourselves. Anything you do that comforts you physically, soothes you emotionally, enriches you mentally, or uplifts you spiritually zeroes in on the appropriate kosha, while simultaneously strengthening and nourishing those connected to it. For example, you get a massage to make your back (physical body) feel better, but you find at the end of the treatment that you also feel happier and more hopeful (the mental or psycho-emotional body, manomayakosha). If instead of seeing a masseuse you visited an acupuncturist, that practitioner would be seeking to alleviate your backache by working with the etheric or energy body. Or perhaps you read the classic *Healing Back Pain: The Mind-Body Connection*, by John E. Sarno, MD, and you're using his protocol to disengage from the emotional and mental imbalance that's beneath the pain—manomayakosha again.

If you're thinking, "Okay, fine, but what does this have to do with feeling younger and aging better?" So much! Your mental body never lay out in the sun with one of those reflectors. Your astral body didn't have x-rays and CT scans and surgeries. Your bliss body didn't subsist for a semester on Coke Zero and cigarettes and call it the dancer diet. It's the physical body that bears the brunt of "ills the flesh is heir to"—sickness, accidents, prescription drugs we needed and others that perhaps we didn't. Our physical body lost sleep because of exams and babies and jet lag. It got food poisoning and the flu, went through menopause and ran four marathons. No wonder a sixty-five-year-old body looks and feels different from one that's twenty-five, expressing as it does forty additional years of showing up for life. But through it all, we have been supported by layers of being, and they support us still.

If you find yourself in a situation in which the physical body is limited by illness or disability, your other vehicles can pick up some of the slack, giving you a richer, fuller life than you might have believed possible. Moreover, the better we treat all our bodies—and this is a pitch-perfect time to start—the healthier and more resilient we will be today and in the future. Breathwork (there's more on this in chapter 7) makes the etheric body purr, while it strengthens our very corporeal respiratory system. Concentration and meditation (chapter 35) are the mental body's mother ship, and yet the physical benefits of meditation include enhanced immunity and normalized blood pressure. Self-study, seeking to know who we really are (chapter 32), nourishes and delights the wisdom body, as well as satisfying the intellect and imbuing us with the recognition that we are, truly, ageless.

I met someone like this a while back at a speaking engagement. This woman handed me a book to sign and as we chatted, she casually mentioned that she was eighty-four. I would have pegged her a well-preserved sixty and my shock evidently showed. She explained, almost apologetically, "It can throw people off that I look the way I do. I haven't had work done, but I grew up in Christian Science and I was taught every day that matter wasn't real and that it had no power over me. I left the church long ago, but those ideas are part of who I am. I seem to be incapable of looking my age or developing the health problems people in their 80s are supposed to get."

What do you think? This is only an anecdote. There will always be outliers who transcend average in terms of IQ, athleticism, wealth, longevity, or something else. It could be that this woman raised on Mary Baker Eddy was simply one of those. Or maybe her mental body was so programmed with the notion that time couldn't touch her that, for eight and a half decades at least, it didn't.

PRACTICES FOR THE PATH

Pick one of your bodies and give it something special today: a hot bath with those Dead Sea salts you got for your birthday; a walk by the water or in the woods; a conversation with someone you adore; a ceremony or ritual that is sacred to you: meditation class, Holy Communion, cleansing the energies in a room with incense or sage. This gift you give yourself will do precisely what it is meant to, even if you're not sure which body (or bodies) you're nurturing.

Part Two

······························

Moving Into Maturity

Chapter 5

Exercise, Physical and Metaphysical

*The body benefits from movement, and the mind benefits
from stillness.*

....

SAKYONG MIPHAM RINPOCHE

In order to age youthfully, there is no substitute for adding activity,
even vigorous activity, to our lives. Yoga doesn't address running and
pumping iron and playing sports, probably because it arose at a time
when daily life called for ample exertion. (For some people, it still does.
When I was in Nepal, I asked a Tibetan refugee how far his childhood village was from the capital, Lhasa. He said, "Not far: thirty days'
walk.") Performing yoga asanas, which we'll address in the next chapter, takes care of some of this, but not all yoga styles focus on building
strength, and almost none substitute for cardio. Both of these, however,
are important throughout life and essential in our later years. That's why
almost everybody exercises regularly, right?

Not right, unfortunately. Our bodies evolved to favor leisure and safeguard the strength and calories our prehistoric forebears needed to sustain
themselves and produce offspring. Some of us—I'm one—seem to have
gotten the evolutionary energy conservation message double. In one of
my earlier books, I dubbed this "Activity Resistance Disorder" (ARD: if it
has initials, insurance may one day pay for treatment). ARD is aversion to

exertion: working out, getting up from the recliner, going for a walk with a friend when meeting for lunch was the other option.

Of course, there can be medical reasons for feeling lethargic—hypothyroidism, anemia, chronic fatigue syndrome, depression, and more. ARD isn't pathology, though; it is more an overwhelming preference for seated pastimes—reading, discussion, theater, lectures, film—and others that aren't quite so high-toned but still compelling: binge-watching, web-browsing, girl talk with a little gossip. Okay, so we're human, but as such, we live in bodies that are designed to move.

As a young person, I was overweight (well, between diets) and already suffering from ARD (undiagnosed since I hadn't invented it yet). When I learned about *hatha yoga*, the now well-known exercise aspect of yoga, it appealed to me immediately. First off, it valued moving slowly and mindfully. (Not all contemporary versions are slow—we'll go into detail on that in the next chapter—but all require paying attention. That's what makes them yoga.) Better still for me, a kid who had once written to a pen pal that I wanted to be a mystic when I grew up, was that yoga said I could bring my soul along. Mrs. Pusateri never mentioned that in gym class.

But before we get into *asanas*, yoga postures, in chapter 6, let's explore the simple wonder of movement itself from a spiritual point of view. We see it in Michelangelo's David, in da Vinci's anatomical sketches, and in Indian and Tibetan renderings of enlightened beings: the persistent concept that strength and beauty are part of the divine design of the human form. Allowing for diversity of body types (remember the doshas: delicate vata, muscular pitta, curvy kapha) and differences in physical ableness, we can strive to express the potential for strength and beauty that each of us possesses now.

The first step is to appreciate your body as it is this minute and trust its God-given ability to add more fitness, grace, and elegance at any age. This will almost certainly require either getting up or lifting something, but it's so worth it. Researchers love putting oldsters on weight-training regimens and report time and again how these subjects defy the odds and build muscle, even in their eighties and nineties when frailty seems to lurk around every couch.

It wasn't these studies, however, that convinced my ARD to take a hike. That came from the bestselling books *Younger Next Year* and *Younger Next Year for Women*, by Chris Crowley and Henry S. Lodge, MD. Dr. Lodge masterfully explains in both volumes that, in addition to building muscle and bone, fending off depression and keeping the ticker ticking, physical exercise alerts the brain through hard-wired neurological circuitry that *we're still worth taking care of.* When we are mobile, the message gets out that mounting an immune response or secreting a helpful hormone is worth doing because an active person is a viable person. The one on the sofa (or, in an earlier era, crouched in a winter cave) is on the way out and not worth the bother.

We know that at any age the body requires cardiovascular exercise (this is what we used to call aerobics: continuous movement, such as walking or running within your training heart rate range), resistance exercise (training with weights and/or weight machines, resistance bands, or your own body weight), and stretching to maintain flexibility. Current physical activity guidelines call for a minimum of 150 minutes of moderate-intensity cardio each week, easily broken into five thirty-minute sessions. Add to this at least two thirty-minute weight training sessions with forty-eight to seventy-two hours between them for recuperation, and stretching after each aerobic or resistance training session. Of course, yoga is without equal for flexibility, and many postures build bone and muscle strength, as well.

Vinyasa yoga sessions (flow styles that keep you moving) may even count as cardio, although it is generally easier on older bodies to rev up the heart rate with swimming, dancing, cycling, or walking at a steady clip, and utilize asana practice for its unique benefits, detailed in the following chapter. But whether you are performing asana or engaged in some other movement, start to see regular exercise as a sacred trust.

The body is a gift to care for and it was engineered to move. Include your spiritual self in the exercise you do already. You can recite affirmations such as "I am healthy and strong" or "Thy will be done" while you're on the treadmill; or you can walk or ride your bike outside with the commitment to see wonder wherever you look. Wear a t-shirt that says, "Heavily Meditated" or "Change Your Energy, Change Your Life."

Most of us grew up with clear distinctions around which activities were physical and which were spiritual: there was soccer practice and Sunday school, and those two weren't meeting any time soon. When yoga hit our hemisphere full force, we were met with the novel notion that physical culture and soul maintenance could take place at the same hour in the same room. That also happens with tai chi, sacred dance, aerial yoga, and Gyrotonics, a bliss-awakening system that involves rhythmic, rotational movements and innovative equipment. In fact, any movement can bring us to that in-the-moment state where the spiritual experience lies.

Adventure sports and similarly challenging activities shine here. We love it when we read about somebody skydiving for the first time on their 80th birthday. We may never do that, but realizing somebody did gives us a hint of the pleasure.

Good old runner's high results when this mental focus meets with endorphins, the feel-good chemicals the body produces in response to even moderate exercise. Becoming lost in dance brings on elation that doesn't crash later like a sugar rush or caffeine buzz. This means that even someone with ARD like me—and maybe you—can get a joy jolt from doing what we used to dread. And there is always the after-it's-over triumph, knowing that you've done something terrific for yourself. Call it instant karma or just desserts, it's yours for simply going through the motions.

PRACTICES FOR THE PATH

Take a fresh stand on sitting. Voluminous research suggests that long periods in a chair can predispose people to an assortment of ills, including type 2 diabetes, hypertension, heart failure, and even some types of cancer. To counteract this, we can first sit better. Lounging, leaning, and slumping are part of the problem. When we sit upright using our back muscles, we counteract many of sitting's ill-effects.

We can also sit less. Maybe you will buy a treadmill desk, or simply set some rules, i.e., to take phone calls and Zoom meetings only while on your feet, or to stand on the bus or subway, even when seats are available. I set an alarm for five minutes before every hour to remind me to unseat myself and do something: walk, tidy up, give a treat to my dog. I will never be an athlete, but Martha Graham, mother of modern dance, said that with the dedicated practice of anything, "One becomes. . .an athlete of God."

Chapter 6

Asana: The Proof Is in the Postures

Yoga is not about touching your toes. It's about what you learn on the way down.

....

DR. JIGAR GOR

As just discussed, movement is potent. Done with a modicum of good sense, it promotes health and, when we give it half a chance, it promotes glee. Hatha yoga, performance of yoga's physical postures or asanas, is movement 2.0. Exercise elevated. Physical fitness that also cultivates the soul. But do remember that even though we talk about yoga class and yoga pants, the physical part of yoga is but a minute aspect of its totality. In his Yoga Sutras, when Patanjali names asana as one of yoga's eight limbs, he defines it as an "easy, relaxed position," one conducive to concentration, meditation, and connection. How, then, did we get to sticky mats, the oxymoron of "competitive yoga," and, according to *Fortune Business Insights*, a global yoga clothing market projected at nearly $47 billion per annum by 2030?

Patanjali penned his sutras, "threads," threads of wisdom, sometime between 200 BCE and 200 CE. The first writings on yoga asanas, as we think of them today, came with the publication of Hatha Yoga Pradipika in 1350. No mere medieval fitness manual, this volume by the Nath Yogi Swatmarama is serious scripture. In it, bodily postures and breath control are used to unblock energy channels (called *nadis* in yoga, meridians in Traditional Chinese Medicine), along with cleansing, purification practices, and dietary guidance to achieve the goal of all yoga, Self-realization.

Nowadays, people are more likely to approach asana practice for health maintenance or stress management. It can come through on both. The postures are designed to affect not only muscles but organs and glands as well. Mrs. Pusateri's jumping jacks and burpees could never claim that.

Classics like downward dog and child's pose help the lymphatic system perform its job of detoxification. The thymus gland, essential for strong immunity and known to shrink with age, is stimulated by bridge pose. Any inversion posture (heart above head, as in headstand, shoulder stand, or legs up the wall) stimulates the pituitary; these poses are also traditionally touted for tightening and rejuvenating facial skin and preventing hair loss. Full forward bend, bow, locust, and triangle pose all aid digestion. If constipation is troubling, look to the various twisting moves, as well as cobra, child's pose, and wind-relieving pose.

Asanas also act to heal emotions. Bow, bridge, camel, cat, crescent moon, mountain, and corpse pose are antidotes to fear. To relieve anger, try pigeon pose, boat, camel, fish, shoulder stand. For overthinking, look to the cow, downward dog, full forward bend, legs up the wall, and tree pose. When you could use more patience, patiently practice cobra, warrior I and II, chair pose, child's pose. If you are new to yoga and these names are unfamiliar, rest assured that they are all basic and will show up in just about any class in town or online.

There is an array of asana styles to choose from, systems adapted, revised, modified, and created in the images of numerous teachers. All include some blend of postures and breathwork. Perhaps a third incorporate meditation, and a quarter call for the full yogic lifestyle we explore in this book. See the following for a sampling of the many styles your search might uncover.

VARIETIES OF YOGIC EXPERIENCE

- *Hatha:* This is both the catch-all term for physical yoga, as well a style unto itself. While passed down through centuries, it can be thought of today as "Sivananda lineage," from Sri Swami Sivananada, a twentieth-century medical doctor turned yogi. (Classes at a Sivananda center, if there is one in your area, are excellent, and include all aspects of a yogic lifestyle.) Hatha yoga movements are slow, focusing the mind, and postures are held, strengthening the body. Relaxation between postures gives the body time to appropriate the benefits. Pranayama is part of every class. Hatha yoga is suitable for all ages, but you'll need to be able to get on and off the floor.

- *Integral Yoga* was developed by one of Sri Sivananda's devotees, Swami Satchidananda, who came to the U.S. in 1965. The asana practice is hatha, and the other elements of yoga—meditation, chanting, selfless service, yogic diet—are included, as well. Level 1 classes are ideal for beginners in midlife and beyond, and Gentle Yoga classes and other accessible alternatives, as well as advanced classes and courses on various aspects of yoga philosophy, are also available at Integral Yoga centers and through their online classes.

- *Vinyasa,* or *flow yoga,* has overshot hatha yoga in popularity and availability. This lineage came to the West via K. Pattabhi Jois in the 1970s. In contrast to hatha yoga's static poses, vinyasa is about movement synchronized with breath. Some classes are not for beginners; if you want one that is, look for the phrase "slow flow."

- *Ashtanga,* also from Pattabhi Jois, is an especially energetic style of vinyasa. Ashtanga means "eight limbs," the full spectrum of yoga philosophy and practice, but an ashtanga class is a rigorous workout based on a pre-set series of postures performed in the same order. If you are reasonably fit, not dealing with arthritis or injuries, and you like a challenge, this may be your bailiwick. (If the class is called *Mysore,* you'll be doing the same series of postures at your own pace, with the guidance of a teacher.)

- *Power yoga,* founded by Bryan Kest, Baron Baptiste, and Beryl Bender Birch, grew from ashtanga and is equally athletic but does not stick to the standard ashtanga poses. While a great way to gain both strength and fitness, this style may best be saved until you've mastered another yoga genre and learned the basic postures.

- *Iyengar Yoga* starts with the genius of its developer, B.K.S. Iyengar, who taught that the better you do the pose, the better it is for you. A high value is placed on anatomically informed alignment, often with the aid of props. Most mid-lifers and seniors can easily start with this system. In fact, it is used by medical doctors, such as New York City physiatrist Loren Fishman, MD, in the prevention and treatment of osteoarthritis, osteoporosis, sciatica, and certain injuries. (Dr. Fishman has a great story of arriving in India with his fresh undergraduate degree in philosophy from Oxford. He knocked on the door of the exalted teacher, woke him up, and spent a year there learning yoga. Medical school followed, at Sri Iyengar's urging.)

- *Jivamukti Yoga*, co-founded by Sharon Gannon, writer of this book's foreword, offers a variety of yoga practices including but not limited to vinyasa, basic alignment classes, restorative classes, and its own meditation practice. Jivamukti's five foundational tenets are *ahimsa* (nonviolence, emphasizing veganism), *bhakti* (devotion to God), *dhyana* (meditation), *nada* (music), and *shastra* (scripture).

- *Kundalini yoga* is a powerful, breath-based system with the goal of bringing forth the dormant spiritual energy called kundalini, the awakening of which opens the chakras. A kundalini class will have you chanting, singing, breathing (heavily at times), and performing postures that test endurance. Those with breathing issues, impaired balance, or joint pain should proceed with caution.

- *Anusara* teaches a hatha yoga asana style with emphasis on correct body alignment and a heart-oriented philosophy committed to the idea that life is good. While the poses can get sophisticated, they are explained well and demonstrated, and teachers are trained to work with each student as an individual.

- *Hot yoga* (sometimes called *Bikram* for the system's founder, Bikram Choudhury) is a series of classic asanas performed in a room that's 90 to 108 degrees Fahrenheit. The heat warms muscles, allowing for more flexibility, and the detox effect from perspiring is its own kind of high. Adherents cite fat loss, muscle growth, and increased stamina. This may be too taxing for someone not already in shape; facial redness that doesn't easily abate ("Bikram rosacea," my dermatologist called it) is another caveat.

- *Chair yoga*: While excellent for seniors, someone rehabbing an injury, or anyone who has difficulty standing or getting up from the floor, a well-taught chair yoga class can provide a real workout. Also, check out "accessible yoga," brought to the fore by Jivana Heyman, author of *Accessible Yoga: Poses and Practices for Every Body*. Whether via chair yoga, bed yoga, or hybrid experiences, this system is dedicated to making yoga accessible to everyone, regardless of age, ableness, or history.

- *Restorative* classes involve passive stretching and constructive rest, bolstered by bolsters, blocks, and blankets to enable fully supported yoga poses held for five or six minutes each. The only physical requirement is that you can make it to the floor. The only psychological requirement is that you're okay with ecstasy. (*Yin yoga* is a specialized type of restorative class, also heavenly.)

If your go-to style isn't in this listing, or if you love one of those cited and think I didn't make it sound sufficiently splendid, my apologies—and congratulations on finding the asana practice of your dreams. (If you want to know what I do, Integral Yoga is the lineage closest to my heart and I take two classes a week. On two other mornings, I lead a hatha-style class in our condo building.)

Yoga's benefits are legendary and studies underscore some of these, including gains in both strength and flexibility, and improvements in balance, stress response, cardiovascular function, blood pressure, cholesterol, and arterial stiffness. Properly instructed and regularly performed, yoga has been shown to increase bone density in older women by one percent per year. One controlled trial looked at eighty-one kundalini yoga students with mild cognitive impairment and showed both short-and-long-term improvements in executive functioning, as well as fewer symptoms of depression and anxiety.

When you talk with people in midlife and past it who practice regularly, they will tell you that yoga is youthening. Bringing consciousness to bear on the body as a whole makes them feel beautiful, sexy even. Because there comes a point at which lean muscle mass is worth more than money, gaining it through yoga is like winning the lottery. Senior yoga practitioners report a newfound ease of movement and have little to contribute to peers' conversations about aches and pains.

On the other hand, people can and do get injured in yoga. If you are starting out, be realistic about your level of fitness, any health concerns or past injuries you need to run by your doctor, and the state of your joints. Knees—the meniscus, specifically—can be vulnerable in yoga, especially if you attempt to sit in lotus or half-lotus pose, or a low-kneeling position (if your kneecaps are sensitive, it can help to use a folded blanket to protect them, and elevate your hips with a block). If you have osteoporosis or osteopenia, refrain from repeated rounding of the back in forward bends: bend from the hips instead (and check out *Yoga for Osteoporosis*, by Loren Fishman, MD). It doesn't matter what the other people in class are doing: look out for yourself.

If you suffer from weak eye capillaries or uncontrolled hypertension, if you have had a stroke or injured your neck, several of the inversion postures—headstand, shoulder stand, fish, plough—are almost certainly contraindicated; stick with legs up the wall until you check with your doctor, physical therapist, or yoga therapist. (Yoga therapists are yoga instructors who have taken 800 additional hours of training in applying yoga principles and practices to improving the health and well-being of individual and small-group clients.)

I deal with old injuries from running, a tumble off a bike, and a couple of car accidents. The closest I've come to a serious yoga injury was a partial meniscus tear sustained in a meditation class of all places, because the teacher wanted us to sit between our feet in a pose called *virasana*, lovely for someone without touchy knees. The little voice that is annoyingly accurate whispered, "Not for you," but I have American competitiveness, a quality best left outside the yoga room, and did it anyway. I have found that a great many yoga moves rehab and strengthen my once assaulted areas. Some other postures can be modified or I just don't do them anymore. There are plenty left.

PRACTICES FOR THE PATH

Adapt an appropriate and appealing asana routine for yourself. I am a big believer in having an in-person teacher, especially if you qualify for senior discounts. If, however, the only classes near you are a style that doesn't feel right, take to the internet. Watch classes of various lineages, try a few—carefully—and see what resonates. Start with one or two each week and practice in between about ten minutes a day, either upon arising, after work, or at bedtime. (Robust activity at night can keep you up, but something gentle—forward bend, cobra, a twist, child's pose, and few minutes of legs up the wall—should help you sleep well and awaken without stiffness.)

Chapter 7

Pranayama: A Breath of Fresh Air

Pranayama is a vital part of daily self-care in ayurveda.
It supports deep cleansing of our mind and the reset of the
autonomic nervous system.

....

RICHARD A. MASLA, AYURVEDIC PRACTITIONER

In yoga, pranayama, breathwork, is central to both physical healing and spiritual observance. It often comes at the end of a yoga class but is far from an afterthought. While different techniques have different aims, the downtempo, deep-breathing exercises that dominate the airy lexicon of yoga slow the heart rate, relax the nervous system, and counter stress. It works on the outside—increased oxygen is a recognized rejuvenator for the skin—and also deep within, yielding additional *prana*, vital energy. A pulmonologist can't measure this with a spirometer, but any martial artist or acupuncturist knows it as *ch'i*. Physicist Max Planck, the developer of quantum theory, described it as a "conscious and intelligent, non-visible, living energy force."

According to yoga, this vital essence flows through nadis, those channels mentioned earlier, the way blood flows through veins. It is lack of prana that keeps a roasted seed from sprouting, and a deficiency of it can keep us from thriving. Insufficient prana may be at the root of fatigue, "stuckness," negativity, digestive upsets, and soreness that can't be blamed on being over the hill or having just climbed one.

Before we get to formal pranayama, let's consider breathing itself, the most essential life activity. People can fast on water only for a month or longer, and survive even without water for at least three days. For oxygen: three minutes. In ordinary life, we don't even have to think about it: our bodies breathe for us. Unfortunately, we do not always breathe the best air. Thank goodness cigarette smoking is on its way out, in this country anyway, but people of my generation were subjected to a lot of those toxic fumes, even if we never smoked. So, we do what we can today:

- Open the windows. Even city air is cleaner than indoor air. Sleep with some fresh air coming into your bedroom and air out every room half an hour a day, preferably in the morning.
- Invest in the best air cleaner you can afford to help clear pollutants and particulate matter that can irritate your lungs.
- Walk whenever possible and get bona fide aerobic exercise at least four days a week. Strength training and strength-building yoga asanas can also shore up the lungs.
- Drink green tea (and matcha, powdered green tea) which has been shown to protect lungs from smoke inhalation and even inhibit the formation of scar tissue.
- Load up on the anti-inflammatory all-stars: berries, leafy greens, turmeric (with black pepper for improved absorption), and cacao.
- Use essential oils, such as frankincense, eucalyptus, rosemary, or a blend such as doTerra's "Breathe," to make breathing easier. These oils are concentrated and potent: just a few drops with water in an oil diffuser or tea-light burner should do the trick, or put those drops on your grandma's hanky and inhale nostalgically.
- If you cook with gas, switch on the vent fan before you turn on a burner. If you can't switch to an electric stove, use your Instant Pot, slow cooker, and electric wok or skillet as much as you can.

And learn pranayama, prescribed as regularly in ayurveda for health maintenance as it is taught in yoga for spiritual growth. Western science has come onboard, too, determining that controlled breathing can support lung function, brain function, and blood pressure regulation. Additionally, slow, deep breathing is a stress-zapper extraordinaire, slowing the heart rate and replacing the sympathetic nervous system's fight, flight, or flee hormones with the tend and befriend (or rest and digest) hormones of the parasympathetic. Results include sharper focus and deeper sleep.

Pranayama is performed two ways, first, as breath synchronized with postures. The general rule here is to inhale on the uplift, the backbend, the opening, and exhale when lowering arms, bending forward, letting go. Then there is pranayama as a freestanding practice. The foundational breath is yogic three-part breathing (*dirgha swasam*), which trains a new practitioner to breathe more fully by allowing the abdomen to expand, then the diaphragm, and finally the chest, with each slow inhalation through the nose. Exhaling, also through the nose unless you're doing a special variation, is equally slow and in the opposite order.

Another popular technique is *kapalabhati*, the bellows breath. Contraindicated in active heart disease but long touted as a preventive for it, this technique involves rapid exhalations, forcefully pressing in the abdomen with each one. This is a morning breath, an energizer. In contrast, another popular standard, *nadi shodhana*, alternate nostril breathing, is the perfect prelude to meditation or sleep, and is also said to balance the left and right hemispheres of the brain.

Like so much of yoga, pranayama is both therapeutically sound and metaphysically meaningful. One of Patanjali's eight limbs of yoga, it has as its first function to calm the disturbances of the mind, eventually enabling us to control (*yama*) the life force energy (*prana*) and unite the individual with the inner divinity. I trust you are spotting a theme here. Yoga, including pranayama, is a Big Picture process. But between here and enlightenment, its techniques give us better odds for good health and extended youthfulness. Win-win.

PRACTICES FOR THE PATH

Treat yourself to the ten-part pranayama course on YouTube from the Sivananda Yoga Center in the southeastern Indian city of Gurgaon (now Gurugram). Just search "Sivananda Pranayama Series." If you have any lung issues, such as asthma or COPD, check with your healthcare provider before starting a breathing practice. If you can't keep up with the pace of instruction, simply don't. One of the most yogic things you can do is let go of the ego and move at a pace that is appropriate for you.

Part Three

Eating Peacefully

Chapter 8

Yoga's Vegetarian Heritage

*Food affects the mind. For the practice of any kind of yoga,
vegetarianism is absolutely necessary since it makes the
mind more pure and harmonious.*

....

BHAGAVAN SRI RAMANA MAHARSHI

I resonated with the word "vegetarian" the first time I heard it. I had
brought the "Four Food Groups" home from first grade. "Humph," said
Dede, my eclectically spiritual, sixty-something nanny. "There are some
people who never eat any meat. They're called vegetarians." I wasn't sure
why, but I liked them.

And five years later on an airplane, I met one. An Indian man was
seated next to me and the flight attendant apologized that his vegetarian meal had not made it onboard. "But I'll tell you what I can do," she
told him, her lilting voice evincing both her Southern roots and TWA
inculcation. "I'll just take your tray, remove the chicken-fried steak, and
bring back everything else for you to enjoy." He thanked her but refused,
saying that he would eat after landing. I couldn't believe it. This man
would voluntarily *starve* for hours in order to have nothing to do with
the slaughter of an animal. That was impressive.

I made some attempts at going veg in my early teens, but it was
yoga that finally got me there. All the books I read simply assumed that
anyone serious about yoga would stop eating meat. For one thing, you
need a reasonably clean, pure body to make progress on the spiritual
path. This comes from food with its life force intact. It is taught that

meditation is enhanced by refraining from consumption of meat, fish, and eggs. And because all living beings want to stay alive, experience pleasure and avoid pain, it is ethically and karmically counterproductive to interfere with their life, liberty, and pursuit of happiness.

For all these reasons, yoga has been vegetarian for about as long as it's been yoga. In Patanjali's Sutras, ahimsa, non-harming, is the first moral precept. We will go into detail about ahimsa when we look at the *yamas* (ways to behave ethically in relation to others) and *niyamas* (ways to behave ethically in relation to ourselves). Ahimsa is in the first category. Traditionally, no student was allowed to study with a respected teacher or guru until they demonstrated mastery of these character-building teachings.

The late Professor Rynn Berry, author of *Food for the Gods: Vegetarianism and the World's Religions*, used to share this allegory. "Let's say you're a true yogi, imbued in ahimsa," he would start out, "and on a hike in the woods you clearly see a handsome buck run off to the west. Then a hunter happens by and asks you which way the deer went. As a yogi, you're supposed to tell the truth, but ahimsa is the highest teaching, so you can blamelessly assure the hunter that the deer went east. If your prevarication isn't sufficiently convincing, you could steal that hunter's arrows or bow. Of course, as a yogi you've mastered the precept of non-stealing, but ahimsa, saving the life of the dear, is the highest teaching. And if even that doesn't work, you can turn from the sacred teaching of brahmacharya, sexual purity, and seduce the hunter if doing so would save the deer. Ahimsa, remember, is the highest teaching."

Berry always got a chuckle from his audience on the seduction part, and no yoga student who heard the story ever forgot it. The teaching is that to do violence, or cause someone else to injure or kill another being, opposes spiritual principles and hampers spiritual progress. And then there is the oneness concept, powerfully stated by Australian philanthropist Philip Wollen when he said: "When we suffer, we suffer as equals. In their capacity to suffer, a dog is a pig, is a cow, is a boy."

Always alert to interconnection, the yogis of yore also recognized how a peace-promoting diet was inherently health promoting. They determined that consumption of vegetables, fruits, legumes, whole grains, nuts and seeds, and dairy products, without meat, fish, or eggs, would aid this. Even though traditional teachings champion the use of dairy, there are plenty of reasons in the twenty-first century to steer clear of it (see chapters 9 and 24). With that sole difference, these suggestions from antiquity are eerily in keeping with current, cutting-edge recommendations in lifestyle medicine. We will delve into this further, but for now I will share something I was told early on. I'd returned from London and Stella's tutelage and was taking asana classes at the YWCA in Kansas City. "Don't bother changing your diet," the instructor told our class. "Yoga will change your diet." For me, it already had.

PRACTICES FOR THE PATH

Catch a veggie movie. The ninety-minute documentary, *A Prayer for Compassion*, follows filmmaker Thomas Jackson on his exploration of food choices and spirituality in many of the world's faith traditions. An absorbing chunk of the film takes place in India. As of this writing, you can watch it for free at www.tinyurl.com/aprayerforcompassion.

Chapter 9

Today's Plant-Based Revolution

Whole plant food is the living language of the sun,
energetically informing and nurturing
the subtle substance of body and soul. It can help you
gracefully embrace the wisdom,
power, and divinity that operates within.

....

FRANK SABATINO, DC, PHD

Looking out for your life and health is important, not because there is nothing beyond this life—according to yogic teachings, there's lots and lots—but because you are here for a purpose. What you can learn, accomplish, and contribute while in a physical body is unique and valuable, and far too many people have, or will, cut their productive lives short because of the Standard American Diet (SAD).

Coronary heart disease kills more people, all genders, in developed countries than anything else. Having it was once viewed as a sure death sentence, but in the 1980s a young internist and yogi, Dean Ornish, MD, showed that even severe coronary disease could be reversed with a low-fat, plant-based diet, asana practice, walking, meditation, and group support. These revolutionary findings were replicated by Caldwell Esselstyn, Jr., MD, at the Cleveland Clinic using only the diet. Since then, this same way of eating, widely known as "whole food plant-based" (WFPB) has been shown to reverse type 2 diabetes and play a role in the prevention and treatment of several cancers (notably colon, breast, and prostate), multiple sclerosis and other autoimmune disorders, and Alzheimer's.

> ## "I GOT 99 PROBLEMS, BUT PROTEIN AIN'T ONE OF THEM."
> ### —Torre Washington, a plant-based bodybuilder
>
> Plant protein is real. It is adequate. And it won't tax your kidneys or promote the growth of cancer cells the way excess animal protein can. (If you're unfamiliar with the research showing this, investigate the work of nutritional biochemist T. Colin Campbell, PhD, and his books *The China Study* and *Whole*.) All protein comes from plants. Animal foods get theirs secondhand. Plant foods with concentrated protein include beans, other legumes (peas, split peas, peanuts) and soy foods, as well as whole grains such as quinoa. But all the whole foods you're eating—greens, potatoes, the hemp seeds on your oatmeal, the hummus in your pita-pocket—contribute protein.
>
> Like children and pregnant and nursing moms, older adults (65+) have slightly higher protein requirements. To ensure adequacy, eat some concentrated protein food or foods at each meal, and frequently choose one of the higher protein plant milks, such as soy or hemp. Learn more in *Plant Powered Protein: Nutrition Essentials and Dietary Guidelines for All Ages*, by Brenda Davis, RD, Vesanto Melina, MS, RD, and Gary Davis, MBA, P.Ag.

Of course, no diet is the key to immortality. While this one is close to a panacea for coronary heart disease, people get sick and older people get sick more than younger ones. There are myriad causes for illness, and "health-shaming" is a terrible practice, whether aimed at ourselves or someone else. We can do only the best we can. Overwhelmingly, current scientific literature implies that, when it comes to nourishing ourselves, adopting a WFPB diet, or coming very close to that, is doing our best.

When I started on my vegetarian path two decades before the Ornish findings were published, it was viewed as a hippie oddity. Now, insurance carriers including Medicare and Medicaid pay for heart patients to go through the Ornish program. In New York City where I live, a plant-based (that means "plant-exclusive") meal is the lunch and dinner default for patients throughout the public hospital system. Even outpatients who present with heart or vascular disease, type 2 diabetes, and/or obesity can opt for conventional care or a treatment regimen that includes counseling on whole food plant-based nutrition and other health-promoting lifestyle interventions.

CALCIUM WITHOUT THE COW

Countries with the greatest dairy consumption have the highest levels of hip fractures among older people, not the expected opposite. Get your calcium where the cow got hers, from greens. Alphabetically, we can choose from arugula, broccoli, bok choy, Brussels sprouts, chard, collard greens, dandelion greens, escarole, frisée—I had to stop at f or I'd have cheated by saying "garden rocket," another name for arugula. Anyway, you get the picture: even before we reach kale and spinach, leafy greens are cheap and easy calcium all-stars that also protect your heart, skin, vision, and brain. In addition, most nondairy milks are fortified with as much calcium as cow's milk, sometimes fifty percent more. (Read the label; a few brands are not so supplemented.) And blackstrap molasses, if you can come to appreciate the strong taste, is a great source of calcium (and iron).

As alluded to earlier, this way of eating comes very close to the recommendations made by yogis thousands of years ago, differing only in that dairy is excluded. So, what's on the magical menu? Plants! Not the philodendron and mother-in-law's tongue, but vegetables, fruits, whole grains, beans and peas and lentils, nuts and seeds, plus life-and-health-enhancing spices and herbs (more on those in chapter 11). As these foods come to populate the pantry and fridge, they crowd out packaged, processed choices. In a short time, they become so enjoyable that yearnings for the old stuff fade.

I hope you are intrigued and I'm sure you have questions. Here are responses to some common concerns, and there is more information in the boxes:

- *Nobody in my family or social circle eats like this.* That's a pity, but

I will bet some of those folks are at least eating *more plants*; the trend is very strong. But even if you are a lone different-drummer diner, some who might give you a hard time will probably admire you too. Studies have shown that healthy habits are contagious, and yours might catch on. In the meantime, bring a dish to share, answer questions without judgment, and stay out of dietary arguments. If someone is interested in doing what you do, they will seek you out.

- *Why hasn't my doctor brought this up?* Physicians get precious little training in nutrition. Pharma reps have their ear; there are no broccoli reps. Educate yourself and maybe you can educate your doctor. I recommend checking out the American College of Lifestyle Medicine, www.lifestylemedicine.org, and Physicians Committee for Responsible Medicine, www.PCRM.org.

- *But I can't eat gluten (or soy or peanuts).* Not a problem. Being plant-based doesn't mean you have to eat every plant. There are over 4,000 edible ones in North America alone.

- *I tried this once and it didn't work for me.* People have said that about marriage and gone on to fifty years of conjugal contentment. You have to live your own life and make your own choices; I simply ask that you remain open to trying again. You are at a different place now and the benefits of eating plants as we age can be spectacular. In addition, if you customize your choices to your doshic profile, you're way ahead of someone going blind on this.

POPPING IRON

The iron in plant foods is not absorbed as readily as that in red meat, but men and post-menopausal women need less iron than younger women do. In fact, too much can be a factor in heart disease; that's why iron is left out of supplements designed for guys or seniors. Legumes provide iron, especially soybeans, red kidney beans, and chickpeas; so do nuts and seeds (sesame, pumpkin, and flaxseeds; cashews, pine nuts, and almonds), and leafy greens: arugula, kale, bok choy, mustard greens, and collard greens. (Some green leafies, notably spinach and turnip greens, contain oxalates that impede iron absorption. They're good foods, but favor other greens if iron is an issue. Black and green tea also have oxalates and tannins that inhibit iron uptake, so drink tea separately from the meals you are counting on for iron.) Enhance absorption by cooking in a cast-iron pot or eating something rich in vitamin C with your iron-rich food (easy fix: sprinkle on lemon juice or include it in your salad dressing).

The other concern people have as they start to look at food in a new way is how to turn whole grains, beans, nuts, and produce into satisfying meals. Do not stress. This is fun. You can't really mess up this food. Okay, you could undercook the brown rice, and almost nobody's eggless muffins grow those big, round tops, but otherwise, plant-based cuisine is foolproof, so not being much of a cook is not much of a problem.

A SUPPLEMENTARY CONVERSATION

Plant foods are replete with vitamins and minerals; supplements are *supplementary*. The noteworthy exception is vitamin B_{12}, which comes from bacteria. All vegetarians (and all humans over fifty, according to the Academy of Medicine, a division of the National Institutes of Health) need to supplement about 250 micrograms per day or 2,500 micrograms per week. Other supplements to consider are:

Vitamin D: We're designed to get this from sun exposure, but due to latitude, skin-protecting melanin, skin-protecting sunscreen, even showering when we come in from a run in the sun, many of us don't get enough. Depending on your existing levels, which your doctor can measure, you may need to supplement; 1,000 IU is commonly recommended.

Omega-3 fatty acids: While flax, chia, hempseeds, and walnuts provide ALA, an omega-3 fatty acid, some people don't translate that well into its usable forms, EPA and DHA. This is the reason some people take fish oil capsules. But we can leave the fish out of this and take an EPA/DHA supplement made from algae. The generally recommended dose is 250 to 500 milligrams of an EPA/DHA combination.

Some people, in consultation with a doctor or dietitian, also choose to supplement:

- Zinc: It's hard to get in any diet; zinc levels decrease with age; and we need it for immune function and to keep our taste buds sharp so food stays yummy all our lives. There is even evidence that zinc may protect against age-related macular degeneration. The RDA for women is eight milligrams daily, 11 milligrams for men, with 40 as the maximum supplemental dose according to the National Institutes of Health.

- Selenium: A micronutrient that protects against cell damage and infection, and assists with thyroid function. You may choose to supplement *unless* you're a fan of Brazil nuts. Even one Brazil nut a day provides all the selenium you need, and more could be too much. As per the Mayo Clinic, base supplementation amounts on daily recommended intakes of 45 to 55 micrograms for women, 40 to 70 micrograms for men.

- Magnesium: A multi-tasking nutrient essential for bones, nerve function, blood sugar, blood pressure, and to reduce inflammation. Magnesium is found in many unprocessed plant foods: nuts and seeds, beans and tofu, avocado, even dark chocolate. Some people have trouble absorbing it and add a supplement; magnesium glycinate is the form most often recommended. Women over 30 need 330 milligrams daily; the RDA for males is 420 milligrams. All adults are cautioned to cap supplementary magnesium at 350 milligrams per day or less (WebMD.com).

- Vitamin K_2: While vitamin K_1 is abundant in green vegetables, plant eaters who don't consume the Japanese soy food, natto, may fall short on vitamin K_2, essential for bone health and calcium metabolism, glowing skin, a strong heart, and a working brain. The recommended supplemental dose is 100 to 300 micrograms, taken at the same time as a vitamin D_3 supplement. (These often come formulated together.)

- Iodine: Essential to produce thyroid hormones, it's found abundantly in sea vegetables (dulse, alaria, nori, wakame—kelp may have too much iodine). You can also get it from iodized salt, but it's a good idea as we age to let go of most salt to avoid the hypertension that affects one in three Americans. Non-pregnant/lactating adults need about 150 micrograms of iodine daily; a supplementary dose should not exceed this amount.

And even with a great diet rich in greenery, some physicians recommend that women over forty supplement with 500 milligrams of calcium per day. I take a supplement called Complement Essentials which contains all the above nutrients except calcium. Another line of supplements I trust implicitly are those from Joel Fuhrman, MD.

Here's an idea of what I eat in a day, wedding whole plant foods and ayurvedic principles.

Breakfast: An oatmeal parfait is standard: oatmeal topped (or layered) with berries, ground flaxseed and walnuts, wheat germ (rich in spermidine, an age-defying nutrient that supports the liver, heart, and brain), and nondairy yogurt or warm soy or hemp milk. But if the bananas are ripe, I treat myself to some variation of the Indian Chocolate Shake from one of my favorite cookbooks, *The Ayurvedic Vegan Kitchen*, by Talya Lutzger (see box). I was an overweight kid always put on diets, so being able to have a chocolate shake for breakfast makes me feel vindicated, and the warming spices make this a year-round meal. Feel free to change things up: I often use soy milk as a base instead of water, a fresh instead of frozen banana, on or two dates instead of three, and add some pea or Brazil nut protein powder and maybe a handful of cherries.

INDIAN CHOCOLATE SHAKE   Talya Lutzger

Ingredients:

1 frozen banana, cut into 3 or 4 pieces (omit or use half for kapha)

1 tablespoon flaxseeds or chia seeds

3 medjool dates, pitted

1 tablespoon grated fresh ginger

½ teaspoon vanilla bean powder or ½ teaspoon vanilla extract

½ teaspoon chili powder

2 teaspoon ground cinnamon

1 teaspoon ground ginger

½ teaspoon ground cloves

1 tablespoon raw cacao powder, cocoa powder, or carob powder

½ cup raw almonds or raw walnuts

8 to 10 ounces water

Instructions:

1. Put all the ingredients in a blender.
2. Process until smooth, stopping occasionally to scrape down the blender jar.

Lunch (although I think of it as dinner since I follow the ayurvedic edict to make this is the biggest meal of the day): My formula is simple: a grain, a green, and a bean. A starchy vegetable, such as sweet potato or winter squash, can stand in for the grain, as can wholegrain pasta or bread made from sprouted wheat or stone-ground flour. Other veggies can accompany the broccoli or collards, and tofu or lentils can play the legume part. The basics stand firm: having a grain, a green, and a bean makes for a nutrient-dense meal that adapts to steaming or stir-frying, a stew, a soup, a salad (having warm veggies in a salad makes it more comforting to vata dosha), a wrap, or a Buddha bowl with lemon-tahini or cashew ranch dressing. There might also be a fruit appetizer or a fun dessert: avocado-based chocolate mousse, maybe, or apple/berry crisp.

Supper: Supper is often soup. Made ahead and served with crudités and good bread, it's perfect. We like split pea, black bean, and minestrone soup, or chili, which is pretty much soup with attitude. Several evenings a week we're likely to have kitchari, ayurveda's healing soup (or stew, depending on how much liquid you add). You may want to start with this tantalizing recipe from Sarah Kucera, DC, CAP, author of *The Ayurveda Self-Care Handbook.*

HEALING KITCHARI   Sarah Kucera

Ingredients:

1 cup white basmati rice

1 cup yellow mung beans (soaked overnight)

1 tablespoon avocado oil

2 teaspoons mustard seeds

1-inch ginger root, peeled and minced

2 tablespoons ground cumin

1 teaspoon ground turmeric

1 bay leaf

1 teaspoon salt

2 cups (300 g) chopped seasonal vegetables (optional)

Doshic- or seasonal-specific chutneys (optional)

Instructions:

1. Rinse the rice and the soaked mung beans until the water runs clear.

2. Heat the oil in a large pot over medium heat.

3. Add the mustard seeds and slowly stir until you hear the first mustard seed pop. Immediately add the ginger, cumin, turmeric, bay leaf, and salt. Stir slowly for 30 seconds to 1 minute.

4. Add the rice and mung beans to the pot and stir until the oil and spices are distributed evenly.

5. Add 6 cups water and bring to a boil. Reduce to a simmer and cover.

6. Cook, stirring occasionally, for about 45 minutes, or until the rice and mung beans are soft and the water has fully absorbed. If you're adding root vegetables or longer-cooking veggies, add them about 20 minutes into cooking. Toss in any leafy greens about 10 minutes before the end of the cook time.

Notes: The mung beans may start to break apart. If the mixture becomes too dry or starts sticking to the bottom before it is fully cooked, add more water.

To serve, optionally add a spoonful of chutney, or top with sesame seeds, and/or chopped cilantro or parsley, if using.

Dining out on plants is pretty easy, as well. These days most cities have at least one vegan restaurant, and other eateries have at least one vegan entrée option—if not, you can get them to combine side dishes with a result that is often so colorful and appealing, tablemates say, "I wish I'd had that." World cuisines tend to be veg-friendly. Chinese places have all kinds of vegetable and tofu dishes, and rice of course. At a Japanese restaurant, you can order avocado, cucumber, or oshinko sushi, seaweed salad, and miso soup. When you go for Thai food, curries abound, or get vegetable pad Thai without the egg, and ask that fish sauce be left out of whatever you order.

Mexican is easy and fun, with bean burritos and veggie quesadillas topping the list; just ask for no cheese. Ethiopian cuisine is superb and the plant-based options are ample since keeping a meatless Lent is common among Ethiopian Christians. Italian is easy—pasta with tomato sauce or with broccoli, garlic, and olive oil, or risotto, if they can do it sans the cheese. And Indian food comes from a vegetarian culture so the choices are ample and satisfying; stipulate that you would like your dish prepared without ghee or other dairy, and you're good to go.

Plants are powerful healers, and a diet composed of them can be sublimely satisfying and blissfully delicious. It is also an integral part of a yogic lifestyle, embodying ahimsa, self-care, and living lightly on the shimmering blue planet where we just might discover heaven on earth.

PRACTICES FOR THE PATH

If you have questions about food or nutrition, or about a health condition and how food might affect it, and you want your answers to come from the scientific literature translated into language a non-scientist can understand, www.nutritionfacts.org is for you. Michael Greger, MD, author of *How Not to Die*, *How Not to Diet*, and *How Not to Age*, scours medical journal articles related to nutrition, collects the information, and uses it to populate his site with short videos for the rest of us. Subscribe for a daily dose of dietary wisdom, and explore the archives where there is likely to be a video on whatever condition, food, or nutrient you're interested in now.

Chapter 10

Food Over 50: Veering Toward Vata

When diet is correct, medicine is of no need. When diet is incorrect, medicine is of no use.

....

AYURVEDIC PROVERB

As we reach the one-quarter mark of this book, let's focus again on its two-fold purpose: One of these is to appropriate yoga philosophy as a way to age with grace, acceptance, and good humor. The other is to age well in the body you are in and hedge your bets toward greater health by applying the teachings of ayurveda and those aspects of yoga that deal with physical health—postures, breathing, meditation.

Considering all this, chapter 10 is one of the most important in *Age Like a Yogi*. What ayurveda offers the crowded and conflicting discourse on effective aging is the bit of brilliance that vata, one of the three doshas we learned about in chapter 2, comes at us full force after our mid-50s. *If we can manage vata, we can manage aging.* This is huge. Here we'll look at managing vata with food. Our personal prakriti, body type, is what it always was, but when flighty vata starts to have its way with us after menopause or andropause, we can start to see and feel evidence of aging. The good news is that we can appease vata with various dietary and lifestyle adaptations so it causes less mischief.

Warm, soothing, easily digestible foods are all balancing for this dosha. Emphasize soups and stews (cooked on low heat for a long time), hot cereals, freshly baked bread (as opposed to light, dry crackers or rice cakes), and the savory Indian porridge, *kitchari*, introduced in the previous chapter. You can think of this as the comfort-food diet, even allowing for some naturally sweetened desserts, such as rice pudding, stewed apples, berry cobbler. Ginger tea works on vata like a charm, ditto blanched almonds. When you come home on a cold or rainy evening, slip on your fuzzy slippers and fix yourself a mug of warm almond milk with cinnamon and cardamom. With each sip, you'll feel the unsettling vata coldness lift, along with any anxiety or nervousness, as vata moves into its balanced role as a creative, life-enhancing part of you.

Obviously, if your body type is mostly vata *and* you're a person of a certain age, you're likely to notice more vata disruption than someone your age whose prakriti leans toward powerful pitta or contented kapha. But vata creeps up on everybody, and knowing how to keep this airy energy contained can be invaluable. For example, vata-predominant people and those in the vata phase of life are known for having "variable digestion." This means that one evening navy bean soup and zucchini bread can be the nicest little supper, and a week later the same menu could lead to gastric distress. Ayurveda contends that most disease starts with improperly digested food, so tending to even mild abdominal discomfort can be an important preventive measure.

Several years ago, I went to an ayurvedic doctor who diagnosed me with out-of-balance vata and handed me a list of foods, the sanctioned on the left side, the forbidden on the right. Nobody wants someone else making their food choices, and with a history of enforced weight loss diets in childhood and adolescence, I was unimpressed. Besides, on the no-no list were superfoods like kale and broccoli. "But these are so healthy!" I blurted out. "No food is nutritious," she pronounced, "that you cannot digest."

Her statement has stayed with me. Does this mean I'm off kale and broccoli? Not at all, *but* if I notice that a stressful life event, recent travel, or eating out more than usual has caused digestive variability to creep in, I make small but meaningful modifications. Instead of kale salad, I will have steamed kale with a lemon-tahini sauce. The cooking process breaks down fibers for greater digestibility, and the fat in the tahini makes an otherwise very light dish more grounding. For someone dealing with too much of a light dosha, this is a good thing. Juicing and blending can also help. And choosing, for a time at least, split mung dal, baby lentils, and tofu over lima beans and garbanzos can give your digestive apparatus, and vata dosha, a chance to reset.

Poor digestion has become so ubiquitous that it can seem normal. Pepcid and Prilosec, Tums and Gas-X are medicine-cabinet staples. Many young people turn to these, and when we reach the age at which excess vata can cause even a cast-iron GI system to get some rust, these digestive aids seem to become essential, along with Metamucil and prune juice. Ayurveda has a simple solution not sold at the drugstore: *Eat foods suited to your constitution, in amounts your digestive apparatus can handle, prepared in the best way for your system to derive maximum benefit.*

THE SHORTEST DISTANCE BETWEEN YOU AND GINGER PICKLES

While you can find more complex recipes, I make ginger pickles by simply scrubbing a fresh ginger bulb (no need to peel it) and cutting it into coin-sized slices. I put the slices in a small bowl and cover the pickles-to-be with lemon juice, a tiny bit of pink salt, and, optionally, a little turmeric and black pepper, allowing everything to marinate three to four hours. Have a pickle or two thirty minutes before your lunch and dinner, or immediately before if you were thinking of other things half an hour ago. These keep well in the fridge, but I make a fresh batch every week to assure my tummy that I'm looking out for her.

Vata, remember, is comprised of air and ether. It is apt to float off like a hydrogen-filled balloon and take a chunk of your stability with it. Foods that are grounding, warming, soothing, and nourishing, with emphasis on the sweet, savory, and sour tastes, are just what the vaidya (ayurvedic doctor) ordered. There are a few tricks to employ, as well. Most important is to make lunch the day's biggest meal. We will talk more about this when we get into daily routine. Just know for now that agni, the digestive fire, is hottest at high noon. To have a bean burrito with veggies and guacamole at that time can be appropriate and nourishing;

at 7 p.m., it could lead to incomplete digestion and an uncomfortable night. Other helpful hacks include ginger pickle before meals (see sidebar) or chewing a few fennel seeds, a quarter to a half-teaspoon, after eating to both aid digestion and sweeten breath.

Keeping vata in check is about listening to yourself and being aware when you start to feel a little cold, a little restless, a little bloated, a little dry. At these times, hot oatmeal with stewed apples will be more appropriate than overnight oats with grated raw apple. This is a day for soup instead of salad, when pasta with garlicy sautéed veggies and a creamy cashew Alfredo sauce would make a dynamic dinner. As we provide care and safety for vata dosha, we feel safe and cared for too.

PRACTICES FOR THE PATH

Plan a day's menu composed of meals you would enjoy that also pacify vata dosha. This may come in handy during vata season, from the onset of fall through early winter, or any day when you find yourself craving comfort and warmth.

Chapter 11

Spices, Herbs, and Rejuvenation

Ounce for ounce, herbs and spices have more antioxidants than any other food group.

....

MICHAEL GREGER, MD

I used to keep cinnamon, nutmeg, allspice, cardamom, and cloves in the freezer, getting them out in December for Christmas cookies and mulled cider. All that changed when I learned about ayurveda. These spices and their colorful kin, from anise seed to zaatar spice, are now in constant use in my kitchen. Beyond assuring no more boring meals, they are antioxidant powerhouses and, according to ayurveda, great healers and regulators. A Yogi.com article by Julie Bernier states that the medicinal properties of ginger, cumin, turmeric, fennel, and cardamom make them the "5 Must-Have Spices for Yogis."

Spices have intrigued our species for millennia. We're drawn to their brilliant colors, intense aromas, and their ability to transform ordinary food into memorable cuisine. If you've traveled to a part of the world where spices are grown, the sensory spectacle of the marketplaces is etched in your psyche forever. Experiencing the scents and colors of even a local spice market is well worth the trip. If you don't have access to a shop like this, look online for organic spices and herbs from a reputable retailer, such as Frontier Co-op.

In their role as antioxidant overachievers, spices and herbs are intimately related to positive aging. Modern science has deemed credible several theories of aging, and most experts accept that a variety of these are at play. One of them, the oxidative stress theory, suggests that as the body uses oxygen, byproducts of oxidation called free radicals are produced that, over time, can damage cells the way rust damages metal. Antioxidants—in colorful plant foods from blueberries to green leaves to red beans, and in spices most of all—have long been seen as the antidote.

Cloves lead the pack in antioxidants, but cinnamon, cilantro, mint—and parsley, sage, rosemary, and thyme, for that matter—make it well worth sticking our noses into spices—aromatic roots, seeds, and the powders made from them—and culinary herbs: highly flavorful leaves, fresh or dried, used in cooking. Both are prized in ayurveda not simply for their nutritive and free-radical-zapping components but for their ability to stimulate and balance the digestive system. According to ayurveda, excellent digestion is key to excellent health. Here are some of the spices lauded by ayurveda and the dosha(s) that favor each. (Tridoshic means all doshas benefit, but frankly, I'll take any spice any time. If one is not my primary dosha's bff, there is likely to be another in the dish that is.)

- **Cardamom** (tridoshic): A versatile spice equally at home in curries, desserts, and teas, cardamom counteracts stomach acidity, stimulates appetite, eases nausea, alleviates bad breath, and relieves gas and bloating. It has also been used as an aphrodisiac (I'm not sure it worked, but for whoever was trying, I hope it did). Use in curried dishes, rice pudding, bread pudding, cookies, carrot cake, and in stews and soups paired with cumin.

- **Cinnamon** (vata and kapha): A single teaspoon has as much antioxidant power as a full cup of blueberries. It also has anti-inflammatory properties, eases digestion, and may help in the regulation of both blood sugar and cholesterol. Cinnamon can benefit the skin and improve cognitive ability; compounds in it show promise in some studies as a possible treatment for cancers. Paradoxically, the most common variety, cassia cinnamon, contains a mild, natural carcinogen, so Dr. Michael Greger recommends Ceylon (or Sri Lanka) cinnamon. It's my favorite topper for oatmeal or yogurt, but also nice on winter squash and sweet potatoes, in stewed apples—ayurveda's go-to for a light breakfast—or to give an uncanny oomph to chili or cocoa.

- **Coriander** (pitta): The seeds of the cilantro plant, coriander tastes citrusy and adds texture to sauces. It has long been praised in India for its anti-inflammatory properties (coriander oil is even used topically for arthritis relief); it also helps soothe the stomach and relieve bloating. Add to soups, sauces, and curries, lentil dishes, potatoes, pickles.

- **Cumin** (vata and kapha): Used as seeds or ground, cumin may up the activity of digestive enzymes, mitigate symptoms of IBS, and protect against type 2 diabetes. It's for chili, of course, and carrots, beets, tomatoes, cabbage, rice, beans, tofu.

- **Fennel seed** (tridoshic): Not only loaded with powerful anti-oxidants, fennel also contains fiber, folate, calcium, magnesium, potassium, and vitamin C. It is believed to boost immunity, reduce blood pressure, and ease abdominal cramping and spasms. Fennel is also a mild appetite suppressant. It's good with greens, roasted veggies, tomato sauces, soups, salads, pasta.

- **Ginger** (vata benefits most from fresh ginger, kapha from dried): Packed with many active compounds, ginger is used to naturally treat nausea from morning sickness or motion sickness (it has been found to rival Dramamine in effectiveness, with no side effects), and its anti-inflammatory properties help ease muscle and joint pain. It also has a diaphoretic property (causes sweating) and so is used to cleanse and detoxify the body, stimulate circulation, and ease bronchitis and congestion. In its culinary role, ginger shows its stuff in cookies, tea, rice dishes, curries, kitchari, stir-fries.

- **Turmeric** (tridoshic): The "king of spices," turmeric is celebrated for its anti-inflammatory effects and used medicinally as well as in food. It appears to inhibit the growth of fat cells and researchers have suggested that turmeric could play a role in slowing the progression of Alzheimer's disease. In ayurveda, turmeric has long been used to aid digestion, relieve joint

SPICES, HERBS, AND REJUVENATION

discomfort, support liver function, and boost immunity. It's essential for scrambled tofu and you can't make a curry without it. While the flavor is strong if overdone, judicious use can take grain or bean dishes, soups, stews, stir-fries, and sauces from simple to sublime. Enhance absorption with the addition of even a little black pepper and a source of fat.

The ayurvedic pharmacopoeia also contains thousands of herbs used exclusively to prevent and treat disease. There's ashwagandha, for example, lauded for its stress-relieving properties and to improve muscle strength, memory, and immune function; and triphala, a combination of three berries with antioxidant and anti-inflammatory properties, often recommended for digestive issues and constipation. There is even a point at which the medical intersects the magical. This is the realm of the *rasayana* (pronounced rah-SY-ana), the alchemical and life-extension arm of ayurveda, a way to nourish tissues at the deepest level.

Just as yoga starts with ethical precepts, engagement with rasayana begins with instructions on moral rectitude. Self-discipline, civility, and the observation of basic social graces are seen as foundational for deep healing and rejuvenation. Rasayana also incorporates elixirs believed to promote youthfulness and verve into advanced age.

Many herbs are considered rasayanas, and there is an esteemed blend long purported to delay aging: *Chyawanprash*—that middle consonant is sometimes a "v." The word is capitalized, not because it's a brand name, but because legend purports that it was developed in pre-antiquity to preserve the life and health of a sage named Chyawan. It is a blend of a up to fifty herbs—formulations vary—made into a jam, usually with ghee and honey, although vegan versions exist, in both powdered and jam forms. Ever curious researchers have studied Chyawanprash and verified its antioxidant and anti-inflammatory properties, as well as its ability to support immune function. There has also been some promising preliminary research into its benefits for cognitive impairment. I look forward to what this reveals, but I'm already impressed by its reputation through countless generations for helping maintain muscle mass, improve digestion, and boost lagging libido. My thinking is this: if your herbs come from a reputable company and don't interfere with pre-scribed medications, there is something intriguing about a youth potion.

PRACTICES FOR THE PATH

Drinking herbal teas can be a gentle and enjoyable way to reap the benefits of herbs. While some can taste more good-for-you than good, the following ayurvedic staples are both delicious and healing:

- CCF tea: This blend of cumin, coriander, and fennel, some-times called ayurveda's miracle tea, is a specific for digestion. You can purchase it ready-made or mix your own: equal parts of cumin, coriander, and fennel seeds in a glass jar. Boil four cups of water and add one and a half teaspoons of the seed mixture. Allow to steep for five minutes and strain. Put in a thermos and sip throughout the day. Ayurveda recommends sipping herbal tea, or warm or hot water, to stay hydrated and avoid too much drinking with meals, which can dampen the digestive fire.

- Ginger tea: Another digestive aid, ginger tea can be sipped as above or drunk on an empty stomach half an hour before a meal to prime agni, the digestive fire. To make it fresh, scrub a ginger bulb and chop a bit of it—one tablespoon or a little less per cup. Bring to a boil; lower heat; simmer for five to seven minutes. And don't diss tea bags; they work too.

- Licorice tea: To balance all three doshas and satisfy a craving for sweets without resorting to sugar, licorice is a divine des-sert tea. (Avoid this one if you're dealing with heart or kidney disease or high blood pressure.)

- Tulsi (holy basil) tea: Acclaimed as an immune booster, con-gestion reliever, and de-stressor, tulsi is even an anti-microbial sometimes used to help prevent tooth decay. It has a reputa-tion for contributing to beautiful skin and strengthening hair follicles to discourage hair loss. Do not drink during preg-nancy or if you take blood-thinning medication.

More notes:

1. You can buy dosha-specific herbal tea blends (www.mapi.com is one source).

2. If you want to sweeten your tea, use coconut nectar, coconut sugar, jaggery (unrefined cane sugar), or maple syrup. (Ayurveda states that honey becomes toxic when heated.)

3. And what about "real" tea, black or green? Ayurveda is generally not thrilled about these because they are drying and stimulating, especially troublesome to vata dosha. However, the science behind tea, green in particular, is very strong. Substances in tea are known to prevent cognitive decline, support bone health, and lower both cholesterol levels and stroke risk. I often have a lightly steeped Earl Grey chai in the morning or green tea at lunchtime, but not later because afternoon caffeine can lead to less sleep at night.

Chapter 12

Divine Dining

Awaken to the specialness—the sacredness even—that
exists within the everyday act of eating.

....

ELLEN KANNER, AUTHOR OF *FEEDING THE HUNGRY GHOST*

In Indian tradition, food offered first to a deity is call *prasad*. It is believed to be blessed in this way, thereby imparting greater health and vibrance when eaten. In other words, preparing food and partaking of it is meant to be holy. You won't see a yogi eating in a car.

People of all cultures have ways of blessing their food. Saying a sincere table grace has been shown to result in slower eating, better digestion, and a higher degree of gratitude overall, resulting in improvement in everything from mood to chronic pain. While 44 percent of Americans purportedly bless their meals, the act is unlikely to have all these benefits when it's a cursory recitation. But even a simple pause for a minute or two, with genuine gratitude and some deep breaths, can enhance digestion. I also believe it makes the food taste better.

We met the term "rasa" in the previous chapter when we talked about rasayana, but it shows up again as we think about consuming food as a sacred endeavor. Rasa translates as taste, but it means more than taste as perceived by the tongue. It is a way of looking at and eating food that's part celebration, part pharmacology. Rasa even makes its way into aesthetics and is used to describe the "juice" or essence of a creative work.

Moreover, while most dietary instructions start with what not to eat, ayurveda insists that we expand our culinary repertoire with the concept of *shad rasa*, six tastes—sweet, sour, salty, bitter, pungent, and astringent—and including all of them in every midday and evening meal (don't worry about it at breakfast; you just got up). This is a revolutionary way of looking at food choices, and for people who have long viewed eating for health as a thou-shalt-not proposition, it is incredibly liberating.

Taking in all six tastes helps ensure nutritional adequacy and satisfy the body's deep yearning for nourishment, so we're less likely to seek the meaning of life at a bakery. The first three tastes are especially good for vata dosha, which might get out of sorts from late fall to early winter, and in our lives' autumn and winter seasons.

- **The sweet taste** isn't to come from sugar and corn syrup, but from fruit, grains (if you chew and keep chewing a mouthful of rice or wholegrain bread, the starches will break down into sugars and taste sweet), milk (I put nondairy milk in this category, too, even though I choose the ones that are unsweetened), and sweet spices, such as cinnamon, cloves, nutmeg (and allspice that captures the flavors of all three), as well as cardamom, mace, and fennel seed.

- **The sour taste** comes to us through lemon, grapefruit, cheeses (if you haven't tried the nondairy varieties lately, they've become good enough to serve to French people), and unsweetened yogurt: look for cheese and yogurt based on almonds, cashews, or, in the case of yogurt, soy.

- **The salty taste** (I like to call it "savory") can be filed under "a little goes a long way." Packaged foods and restaurant meals usually have way too much salt; so does bread, with a few exceptions, such as Ezekiel 4:9 Low Sodium Sprouted Grain Bread, or what you bake yourself. The various seasoning blends meant to stand in for salt highlight the naturally occurring sodium in celery and other vegetables. Sea vegetables—dulse is my favorite—have naturally occurring sodium, too, along with lots of minerals. You can buy granulated dulse and use it in some instances where you'd otherwise have used salt. Ayurveda does not advise a diet free of added salt for everyone, but many medical professionals do. I have some Himalayan pink salt in my pantry and use it sparingly.

- **The bitter taste** comes in bitter greens like dandelion and collards, and in eggplant, sesame seeds and tahini, dark chocolate, coffee, and the spices turmeric, saffron, cumin, fenugreek, and dill. It is especially beneficial for kapha and pitta types, and during kapha season (late winter through spring) and pitta season (summer and early autumn).

- **The pungent taste** is what most people think of when they hear the word "spicy." It is characteristic of Indian, Thai, Mexican, Szechuan, and Ethiopian cuisines. You'll find this taste in spices, such as black pepper, chiles, ginger, mustard seeds, cardamom, cayenne, cloves, paprika, and asafetida (hing), and in foods including onion, garlic, leeks, mustard greens, and radishes. This taste is especially beneficial for kapha people and during kapha season.

- **The astringent taste** is not known by that name to most people before exploring ayurveda, but when it is explained, we're apt to say, "Okay, I get it." Think about what the following foods have in common: pomegranates, raw apples, unripe bananas, white potatoes, pasta, most beans, popcorn, raw veggies, green and black teas. And then compare these spices: basil, bay leaves, carraway, marjoram, nutmeg, oregano, rosemary. There's a clean dryness to all these, a coolness, and a slight puckery sensation in the mouth. It's subtle, but everybody likes pasta and potatoes, and astringency balances pitta dosha most of all.

Make a game of getting the six tastes into each meal. Here's a sample: a Buddha bowl comprised of rice (sweet), chickpeas (astringent), radicchio (bitter), and arugula (pungent), garnished with a few olives (salty) and topped with a lemon-tahini sauce (sour).

The great gift of a yogic/ayurvedic food style is that even the simplest repast is a creative act, and eating food, digesting it, and assimilating its nutritive properties is a chemical but also an alchemical process. When we talked about the five bodies, we learned that the physical body is the annamaya kosha; that translates as "food sheath." Every meal, then, is a construction job, maintaining and recreating our earthly selves. Building materials can come from the farmers' market or the convenience store. Those of us fortunate enough to have a choice would do well to choose wisely.

In the yogic view, this goes beyond nutrition. What does your food look like? Is it colorful?—colored by nature, of course, not FD&C 1, 3, 5, and the rest. Is it freshly prepared? When using last night's leftovers or batch cooking on the weekend means a homemade meal instead of the drive-thru, it's worth doing. Just know that there is more prana in foods fresh from nature or those you've cooked for the first time. If you are reheating a soup, serve it with some crudités. If the entrée is one you froze last weekend, have a couple of kinds of freshly steamed or sautéed veggies with it.

And whether you are pre-cooking, reheating, or starting from scratch, what's your mood in the kitchen? If you adore cooking, great. You will grace your dishes with love and positive energy. Or maybe you once enjoyed cooking but you're at a been there/done that place with it. I was right around fifty when one day either my husband or my daughter walked in—I don't recall which—and innocently asked, "What's for dinner?" I had to stop myself from blurting out, "Fix your own damn dinner!" I was shocked. I had always seen food prep as a creative outlet, but in that instant, I knew I was done. In my next phase of life, I would need food to be simpler and life to be richer. That is what's happened.

A Sikh friend, adept in kundalini yoga, shared with me long ago that the attitude of the cook is as important to the meal as its nutritional profile. She taught me to stand at the edge of the kitchen and scan my psyche like an ethereal x-ray. If I detected anger, resentment, anxiety, or impatience, I would need to meditate or go outside in the sunlight and gaze at some petunias. Otherwise, my negative attitude would go into the food like an unwanted additive.

Then there's the accessorizing of meals with flowers on the table and lovely dinnerware. (If you are old enough to read this book, you're past saving the good dishes.) A simple place to start is by keeping the table clear, ready to fulfill its purpose of providing the backdrop for nourishment. While there are few phrases more archaic than "dress for dinner," we can at least wash up and wake up for our primary meals. A lovely spritz of rose hydrosol is an ayurvedic suggestion for instantly being here now, all senses engaged, all systems go. Sit and smile, even if you're by yourself. Chew your food (ayurveda says thirty-two times for each bite; I would find the counting tiresome).

Whether at home or out, alone or in company, enjoy the meal and acknowledge its ending. I learned a lovely way to do this from a Protestant friend who visited a Catholic mass. When the priest said, "The mass is ended: go in peace," she adapted that as "The meal is ended; I go in peace," to provide punctuation between eating when it's time to eat and living when it's time to live. Feel free to borrow this. I don't think she'll mind.

PRACTICES FOR THE PATH

Bless your food. If you already have a way to do this, it is the right way. If not, try this: Sit for a few moments with your hands in your lap, palms up, eyes closed. Enjoy a couple of nice, easy breaths. Take a moment to recognize that, in addition to the vital energy you get from breathing, you are about to take in very tangible energy in the form of food. That food got to you via the grace of God, as well as some hard-working farmers, truckers, grocers, and earthworms—not to mention a skillful chef who may very well be you. Bon appétit.

Part Four

·····································

Your Sacred Schedule

Chapter 13

First Thing in the Morning

The ideal time for spiritual practices like meditation and
chanting is Brahma Muhurta.
During this period, sattvic qualities are predominant in
nature. Moreover, the mind
will be clear and the body energetic.

....

MATA AMRITANANDAMAYI, "THE HUGGING SAINT"

Suggested in yoga and integral to ayurveda is the notion that when
we do things is as important as how we do them. Circadian medicine, a relative newcomer on the Western medical landscape, concurs.
Ayurveda insists that nature, including the twenty-four-hour day, is
cyclic and rhythmic. When we understand this and operate within the
natural framework, we'll feel better physically and emotionally.

Morning is so important that it gets a chapter all its own. There is a
pre-sunrise period that yoga calls *Brahma muhurta*, "the Creator's time,"
believed to be ideal for meditation. If you want to pinpoint this time, it
begins at one hour and thirty-six minutes before sunrise and ends forty-eight minutes prior to the sun's coming up. Most of us will say, "That's
ducky for some people, but way too early for me." Fair enough. However,
sleep patterns change with age. A lot of older people fall asleep just fine
but awaken earlier than they'd planned and feel discouraged when this
happens. The realization that being awake during Brahma muhurta is a
grace can make it easier to reframe awakening when the birds do, provided you got to bed on the early side the night before.

Do what you will with pre-dawn meditation, but getting up by 6 a.m. is as close as ayurveda comes to a non-negotiable. You see, the day is governed by those same doshic energies that identify us. When our bodies' rhythms and the day's rhythms are in sync, we tend to move through those days with less effort.

- Vata time is 2 to 6 a.m. (this accounts for some of that very early waking many in the vata stage of life experience) and 2 to 6 p.m.
- Kapha time 6 to 10 a.m. and 6 to 10 p.m.
- Pitta time is 10 to 2 p.m. and 10 to 2 a.m.

If you'll remember, kapha energy tends to be heavy. That's why it is strongly suggested that we rise by 6 a.m. If we go too much further into kapha time, we're likely to awaken sluggish and groggy instead of bright-eyed and ready for the day.

Once we are up, what do we do? There is no shortage of recommendations. If I attempted to accomplish everything I've read or been advised by spiritual teachers and ayurvedic doctors to do "first thing in the morning," it would take until afternoon. I will cover here what I personally see as ayurveda's "Foremost Five," important activities for morning that you would do well to incorporate into your routine, and the time it might take to do them. I'll list additional suggestions in the Practices for the Path at the end of this chapter.

THE FOREMOST FIVE

1. *Splash* (your eyes and face), *swish* (your mouth), and *scrape* (your tongue): five to fifteen minutes. (See sidebar.)

2. *Get some early daylight, ideally paired with a morning walk*: fifteen to thirty minutes. Early morning sun sets our internal clock so we have more energy for the day and an up-regulated mood. "When sunlight enters your eyes, your entire brain lights up," says Jacob Liberman, MD, author of *Luminous Life: How the Science of Light Unlocks the Art of Living*. Barring extenuating circumstances (a 4 p.m. espresso would

be extenuating), early exposure to natural light will improve sleep quality that night. On cloudy days, one of those special lights for Seasonal Affective Disorder can substitute. In the dark of winter, you wouldn't be overdoing it to take an early morning walk *and* spend fifteen minutes near a light therapy lamp (they are inexpensive and easy to find online).

3. *Drink warm water with lemon*: five to ten minutes. We dehydrate overnight. Ayurveda's remedy is to drink twelve to sixteen ounces of water with some fresh lemon. This both rehydrates thirsty tissues and stimulates peristalsis in the gut, encouraging a morning bowel movement. Should you find warm water unpleasant, hot is fine; so is room temperature. If you are concerned about tooth enamel erosion from the lemon juice, rinsing after and waiting at least fifteen minutes before brushing your teeth should protect against that, or ditch the lemon and drink plain water or ginger tea. Either way, this is your big gulp. During the day, keep a thermos nearby for frequent sipping.

4. Enjoy *abhyanga*, warm oil massage: five minutes to apply with an optional twenty more to allow the oil to soak in. (See sidebar.)

5. Practice your yoga for twenty to sixty minutes. Include asana, pranayama, and meditation.

SPLASH, SWISH, AND SCRAPE

Splash your eyes a few times with cool water to remove any dirt or discharge that has built up overnight, and since one seat of fiery Pitta dosha is the eyes, the coolness benefits them. Then splash your entire face—seven times for the seven chakras, some folks say—to wake you up, add luminosity to your skin through increased blood flow, and lessen early a.m. puffiness.

Swish your mouth with about a tablespoon of cold-pressed sesame (that's traditional) or olive or coconut oil. This is called oil pulling. It generates antioxidants that eradicate unwanted microorganisms, and the fatty membrane encasing single-cell bacteria in the mouth attaches to the oil to be expelled along with it. The result: stronger (even whiter) teeth and healthier gums—a very big deal since oral bacteria can affect other body systems and even contribute to heart disease.

To do oil pulling, swish the oil around the mouth as you would mouthwash but not as energetically since this is going to take more time: twelve minutes for maximum benefit, but start with three and work up. (Some people multi-task and swish in the shower.) Be careful not to swallow any oil and the toxins it's picked up; spit into a trash receptacle, not down the drain where it could clog pipes; then rinse with pure water to which you have added an (optional) pinch of salt.

Scrape your tongue to remove the *ama*, metabolic debris, that's built up overnight. This is a ten-second detox that freshens breath and keeps your tastebuds up to par. Use a copper or stainless-steel tongue scraper (order online or find at a natural food store or Indian market) to gently remove any build-up, four or five times from back to front, rinsing the scraper in between. Brush and floss after breakfast.

ABHYANGA, WARM OIL MASSAGE

When I think of massage, it is about the strokes, the pressure. This self-massage is different. It's about the oil, *sneha* in Sanskrit, which also means love. This process calms the nerves, lowers blood pressure, makes skin healthier, helps ease joint stiffness and pain, lowers systemic inflammation, and seems to help those who run cold stay warmer.

To do self-abhyanga, slightly warm untoasted sesame oil (or almond if you prefer a lighter texture) in an aromatherapy oil burner or put the oil in a plastic bottle and place that in a mug of hot water to warm it up. A quarter cup of oil is more than enough. Start massaging at the top of your head unless you don't plan to wash your hair; in that case, skip your head but include your face. Sesame oil doesn't tend to clog pores and shouldn't cause breakouts. Obviously, if you are the exception to that, you'll keep it off your face. If not, you may find that this simple oil becomes your favorite moisturizer.

Use long strokes over bones, circular motions around joints and fleshy parts of the body, and spend the most time on your head and feet. If you can, keep the oil on your body for twenty minutes. If you don't have this much time, give it five minutes and shower.

> Important note: *Oil is slippery and if you're at all unsteady, do not do this. And even if you are steady, be careful.* Thoroughly wipe any remaining oil off your feet with a dry towel before stepping into the shower. Wear shower shoes with those sticky pads on the bottom. Take no chances. Oil can also catch fire, so check your dryer setting to be sure you'll be safe drying oily towels there.
>
> Depending on the season—fall and winter are ideal for this—and how you feel, once or twice a week might be all you need, although someone with a lot of vata imbalance could benefit from fitting this in almost every day. In addition, abhyanga, while most often presented as a morning ritual, can be done in the evening before a warm bath.

Doing all this is without doubt a commitment, but those who make it swear that the payoff is well worth the time expenditure. Don't be discouraged by thinking your rejuvenation rests on doing everything every day. If you need to be at your desk by 8:30 a.m. and you like to hit the gym beforehand, maybe all you can do from this list during the week is splash your face, scrape your tongue, meditate for five minutes, and get your water allotment in while on the treadmill. How amazing that you did all that! The least I can do is offer you breakfast.

In ayurveda, breakfast can be light but never skipped. You may be satisfied with only stewed apples, pears, or bananas with spices, or a fresh fruit salad with a couple of pinches of the spice blend, *chat* (sometimes with two a's) *masala*. (You won't believe until you taste it what this sour mango powder with tangy ajwan seeds can do for a bowl of fruit.)

If you need a more substantial breakfast, hot cereal (oatmeal, cream of wheat, roasted rice) with spices and fruit and nut toppings are good. So are root vegetables, such as sweet potato or butternut squash, steamed or roasted and served with chopped dates and walnuts. If your breakfast makes you feel sleepy or groggy, go over all its components and see if there is an item to weed out. Ideally, breakfast will make you feel that you're up for the grandest gift anyone was ever given: one more day.

Ayurveda is bursting with suggestions for ways to love yourself up while some people are still snoozing. You might add one or two of these additional techniques on the occasional morning, or perhaps some lovely Saturday you'll give yourself a spa day and do them all. Note that only the first three are for morning implementation only; the others you can save for evening or some other time.

- **Treat each of your five senses** to something lovely first thing: you might *see* a picture of your family, *touch* your cat's fur, *hear* the birds chirping, *smell* your favorite essential oil, and *taste* a perfect bite of dark chocolate.
- **Experience the sunrise.**
- **Spend twenty minutes with your bare feet touching the earth.**
- **Perform nasya,** a mini ritual of lubricating the nasal passages, considered in ayurveda the "gateway to consciousness." Nasya helps with freer breathing (it's good to do before pranayama), mental clarity, and has traditionally been seen as an aid to vision and vocal quality. Use plain sesame oil or a special nasya oil with helpful herbs. (I like the one from Banyan Botanicals, spiked with brahmi and calamus.) While there are more intense ways to do this, the most accessible is (1) put two or three of drops of oil onto the pad of your little finger, (2) rub it into your right nostril, (3) hold the left nostril shut and sniff to bring the oil further into your nasal passages, (4) repeat on the other side. This is best done an hour before or after showering or exercise, or twenty-four hours before or after nasal cleansing with saltwater and a neti pot (chapter 29).
- **Oil your ears.** Sesame or olive oil works, but again, I like an herb-enhanced ear oil. It's nice to warm the oil slightly by placing the dropper bottle in a mug of warm water for a few minutes. Then drop two to three drops into your right ear by

lying on your left side for a couple of minutes. It should drain out immediately when you sit up or tilt your head to the right. If it doesn't, pull on your earlobe to open the passage. Repeat on the left side. (Notes: 1. Never do ear oiling when a perforated eardrum might be present. 2. Never stick a cotton swab or any other object into your ear.)

Chapter 14

Each Day's Journey into Night

*Many of our most common physical complaints are created
or exacerbated by a modern schedule
at odds with the body's needs.*

....

SUHAS KSHIRSAGAR, MD

Dinacharya is the name given to daily routine, and it covers all twenty-four hours. Morning routine just got its chapter, and in the current one we will look at everything between breakfast and supper.

We instinctively try to time things right. If you lived in an apartment building with a certain amount of hot water and you knew from experience that showering after 7 a.m. would mean initiation into the Polar Bear Club, you would find a way to shower before then. Well, you live in a body with a certain amount of digestive capacity, and whether yours is excellent or sometimes weak, you want to work with it. An important way to do this is to have your heaviest meal at midday because, just like showering when the water is hot, your digestive fire will best perform its vital work when at its peak.

For most of us, this is a different way of doing lunch, and it can take some planning. If you're at home, use a slow cooker to have kitchari, soup, rice and beans (or rice and dal) ready at noontime; or put a casserole you pre-assembled into the oven an hour before your intended luncheon. Another option is to steam a starchy vegetable, a green vegetable, and some pre-cooked beans, and serve with a sauce you have on hand: gingery miso, maybe, or nut-based pesto. While fresh is always best, there are prepared sauces available at natural food stores that are made from excellent ingredients.

If you take your lunch to work, pack something warm and nour-ishing. If you're used to having a little dessert with your evening meal, flip that: have it now instead. Even if you can follow the bigger-mid-day-meal suggestion only partially—i.e., a slightly heavier lunch and a lighter dinner—the benefits will soon speak for themselves. And on the days you're in charge of your schedule, you can rethink "breakfast, lunch, dinner," and consider "breakfast, dinner, supper."

IN THE GOOD OLD SUMMERTIME

A word here on Daylight Saving (British Summer Time in the UK): Most U.S. states and some seventy other countries go through a biannual ritual of moving the clocks forward and back, so that half the time what your watch says and what the sun is doing are in sync, and half the time they aren't. This is no mere inconvenience. At the times when we "change the clocks," hospital admissions increase, and there is a higher incidence of heart attacks and strokes. Anxiety and depression are exacerbated.

These ill effects are more noticeable when we're forced to "spring forward" just as kapha season, with its heaviness and slowness, takes hold. Nature has been proceeding on schedule; we are awakening with the sun after winter's long nights, and then a bureaucratic decision from the mid-twentieth century sends us back to waking in the dark. There is talk in this country about scrapping the current system and hav-ing Daylight Saving all year, so we would never be on sun time. The experts in chronobiology insist that we should indeed get rid of the time changes, but in favor of Standard Time. We're physiologically wired for light mornings and dark nights, and we challenge this to our peril.

So, what do we do? Adapt as best we can. Some adherents of ayurveda shift their time of rising, retiring, and meals to stay with the sun's schedule throughout the year. I just spring forward and fall back and attempt to take better care of myself during the transition times. It is not perfect but good enough.

After the midday meal, you would be wise to consider the long-standing ayurvedic recommendation to take a little stroll outside for ten minutes. This isn't a power walk, just some leisurely meandering to help the digestive process along; it can also help you get through the afternoon without that dreadful slump. If the weather is bad, you could walk on a treadmill at under three miles per hour, or aid your digestion with LSD: lying for those ten minutes with your Left Side Down.

Should you feel droopy at three or four in the afternoon, get up. Get out if you can. Move about. Have some herbal tea (or even weak green tea if you're in a caffeine-or-bust situation). Spritz rose hydrosol on your face. Sit in the sun, with SPF of course, for a five-minute mini meditation. The first ayurvedic physician I ever saw, thirty years ago now, assessed my doshic status and advised licorice tea at 3 p.m., along with a sliver of apple pie. I had never before been prescribed pie. He also suggested something sweet for the soul: a second daily meditation in the late afternoon or early evening.

We will focus on meditation in chapter 35. Suffice it to say for now that if you're someone looking to add a second period of "restful alertness" to your day, the late afternoon is perfect for this. If you work in an office or teach in a classroom with a door you can close, you might stay and meditate there, or fit in your quiet time as soon as you arrive home. Some studies have shown that twenty minutes of meditation refreshes the body as much as two and a half hours of sleep, but without post-nap fogginess. If you're typical, you will notice a little lift, perhaps enough that you'll want to visit friends in the evening rather than collapse in the recliner.

Now it's time for another meal. Timing is everything, of course, so see if you can have your evening meal no later than seven. If you finish in thirty minutes, you will have two and a half hours of digestion time before going to sleep at ten. That's good. If you can eat even a bit earlier and give your body three hours for digestion, better still.

We're talking here about a light meal. "Supper" comes from the same root as "supplement." Soup or kitchari is perfect. So is a small portion of pasta and some steamed or sautéed greens. Or have breakfast for dinner:

oatmeal with berries, seeds, and spices, or scrambled tofu with veggies and a slice of sourdough toast.

A ten-minute stroll, like we talked about after lunch, is also appropriate now. Then, once the dishes are done and the kitchen is presentable—you don't want a dirty kitchen to greet you in the morning—you'll find yourself with a few hours of evening. Ayurveda says that this is actually the start of the day that's coming, because what you do between supper and bedtime—as well as when bedtime is—will have a thoroughgoing effect on how you sleep, how you awaken, and the mood you'll be in when you do. Evening exists for pleasure and winding down. If you want to watch TV, choose a comedy or a heartening biopic. Call a 7 p.m. halt to news consumption. Schedule difficult conversations for daytime. Now, play a board game, check in with someone you'd really like to talk to, read something inspiring, or take a restorative yoga class or a leisurely soak in the tub with whatever scents and extras would make the experience ultra-relaxing.

If possible, have your last hour of waking without screens—no phone, laptop, TV, any of them. Their blue light interferes with production of the melatonin that invites sleep. It helps if you put devices on night mode. You can even buy special glasses to filter out the blue light, but ideally you will simply experience this crucial hour of the day without an electronic sidekick. Charge your devices anywhere except your bedroom. If your phone is your wake-up alarm, try to charge it during the day and keep it on airplane mode at night. Make your room dark, even if that means wearing a sleep mask. If it is practical to sleep with an open window, do so. Before sleep, go over the day just past and if there is anything you missed or anyone you need to contact, make things right with, or reassure, note that. And then tell yourself that the past is over, the present is as it is, and the future has gifts of its own

PRACTICES FOR THE PATH

Ayurveda's gift for better sleep is to massage your feet at bedtime with warm sesame oil, perhaps with the addition of a few drops of some sleep-inducing essential oil, such as lavender, bergamot, or marjoram. Gently heat the oil in a tea-light burner (be sure you blow out the candle) or by immersing a small container of oil in a mug of hot water. Then massage each foot, all parts, giving a little extra attention to any areas of discomfort. Cover with cotton or bamboo socks that don't have a tight band. (Choose the kind with non-slip soles if you're apt to be walking to the bathroom at night.) If you like, you can also massage the oil into your hands and perhaps a bit on your temples. I do this when I am already in bed. After that, I'm seriously out like a light.

Chapter 15

Seasonal Sadhana

Spring passes and one remembers one's innocence. Summer passes and one remembers one's exuberance. Autumn passes and one remembers one's reverence. Winter passes and one remembers one's perseverance.

....

YOKO ONO

Sadhana means spiritual practice and while we're on earth, that practice includes cooperation with nature and her shifting seasons. In this context, ayurveda asks us to think in terms of three seasons rather than four, each governed by one of those ever-present doshas. While local variations in climate and the reality of climate change have some impact, the underlying characteristics of these three seasons still apply, and they do so wherever we find ourselves.

- Late winter and spring are kapha season, when it's likely to be damp and probably still chilly.
- Summer belongs to pitta, bringing with it the challenge of keeping cool without resorting to the frosty foods and iced beverages that, even this time of year, can dampen the digestive fire.
- Fall and early winter are vata time. Since vata goes out of balance more easily than the other doshas, we need to be especially diligent this time of year to keep to a regular schedule, eat warm, nourishing foods, and indulge in a little more quiet and a little more comfort than we might ordinarily allow ourselves.

The first secret to seasonal sadhana is to be aware of the seasons and, if you can, interact with each one consciously and curiously. This requires spending time outdoors, or if you can't get outside, looking out a window. You want to be aware of what season the planet is experiencing in the area where you are because your body/mind complex is experiencing it too. Modern fabrics tend to be multi-seasonal, but the ritual of exchanging summer clothes for winter ones is a simple way to internalize that nature is making an adjustment, we're part of nature, and we acknowledge this by doing some adjusting of our own.

Let's take a trip around the year starting when the planet does, springtime. We will be talking ayurvedic springtime, kapha season, which also includes late winter and whatever post-equinox weeks or months feel like winter where you are. We feel more balanced in this cool, wet season if we provide ourselves with warmth, stimulation, and some dryness. Wear layers. Visit the sauna. Turn on music that makes you dance. Take a spring vacation. When the day is sunny, find reasons to be out in all that kapha-embracing light.

Add kapha-balancing foods to your diet: the antioxidant superstars, berries and cherries; citrus fruits and red bell peppers with all their vitamin C; versatile black beans and zinc-rich pumpkin seeds; as well sprouts, microgreens, and the fresh greenery popping up in your garden and at the farmers' market. In springtime, even fussy vata can handle some of these foods. They should help you avoid seasonal sniffles and the mild depression that can come from all those April showers. And if you picked up a few pounds between November and February, these foods will help you release them without effort.

As summer approaches, we enter pitta season. Most people love it, including elders prone to feeling the cold. Pitta is energizing and motivating. Do you notice how people say, "Have you made plans for summer yet?" and "Will you be getting away this summer?" in a way they simply don't ask about other seasons. It is expected that in summer we are going to *do something*—that's very pitta. The upside is that vata and kapha types will finally warm up (unless ubiquitous air-conditioning interferes). The aches and pains that came with winter and spring often abate, and we're apt to find ourselves passionate about some project or cause.

The downside is, as ever, too much of a good thing: too much heat, too much ambition, and too much effort feed pitta dosha. In summer especially, this can lead to skin eruptions, inflammatory irritations of various sorts, angry outbursts, and indigestion. But wait, doesn't pitta equate to strong digestive fire? Yep, but excess can lead to upset, i.e., heart*burn*. Avoid the negatives and delight in the positives of pitta season by drinking pure coconut water or blended watermelon or cantaloupe, no ice; these are great coolers. It helps to consume traditional summer foods, such as zucchini, cucumber, celery, mint, and mangoes, as well as to exercise early and stay out of the midday sun.

Equally important: *slow down*. I mean, how many summers do we get? How many marvels will you miss if you dash through this one as if you had a million more? Skip some stuff. Look at your calendar and appreciate the empty spaces. You might even schedule in empty space as if it were an appointment, because before you know it, you'll have an appointment with autumn, vata season.

The way ayurveda sees things, vata season starts as summer wanes. There will still be the occasional hot day, or even a warm week, but it is clear from the air in the morning and the produce at the market that things are shifting. If you are in a locale where it's normal to swim outdoors in October, you probably have a month before vata season starts. If, on the other hand, you're somewhere that the kids need hoodies to start school in September, you can presume that vata season has begun. Should you be in a locale with little change in temperature, you will need to pay attention to nature's subtler signals. My mother, who lived in Florida for the second half of her life, told me that, even there, she could "smell the fall."

If you're in your personal vata season (over age fifty-five, more or less), you'd do well to take tender care of your vata side during the autumn and early winter months. Doing so will mean a healthier you, a happier holiday season, and, I fully believe, a slower aging rate during these months than you would have had otherwise.

Because vata is cold, dry, and skittish, you'll want to add warmth, moisture, and stability to your life during this season and during these years. Failing to do this can lead to vata imbalances that show up as digestive distress, feeling chilly even in a warm room, getting tired easily, and having more senior moments. If you notice these little brain lapses and your doctor assures you that, clinically, you're fine, you may be looking at a vata imbalance. This is as common as dirt, because vata is so ungrounded. Keeping it stable is a job, especially in our stimulating modern world that is all but designed to aggravate vata dosha.

So, here's your prescription—a good one for fall and winter at any age and essential when in or approaching act three. *Keep your schedule dependable, your environment on the quiet side, your room and clothing warm enough, and your self-care prioritized.* This is the time to do abhyanga, the warm oil massage we learned in chapter 13, more often, even daily.

Stay closer now than any other time of year to those foods that reduce vata. Review chapter 10, and recommit to an emphasis on comforting, easy-to-digest foods. Think warm and mushy: soup, stew, porridge, puddings, sauces with some substance to them. But even in this season, avoid a thou-shalt-not mindset. Unless it disagrees with you for some reason, no wonderful offering from the plant kingdom is verboten. Just don't overdo the cold, raw, light, dry foods that aggravate vata, and prepare them in a vata-pacifying way: slow-cooked, sautéed, or steamed with the addition of some EVOO, avocado, nuts, seeds, or nut butter. The idea is to stay down to earth, even though you're made of the stuff of stars.

PRACTICES FOR THE PATH

If you're not a regular farmers' market shopper, you would still do well to go once a month. This will give you an evolving idea of how the seasons affect what foods are available in your part of the world. Being around all that seasonal produce is also a great way to embrace the season you're in, and the just-picked freshness of those fruits and veggies means they're brimming with both nutrients and prana, life force energy.

Part Five

The Glow Factor

Chapter 16

Oh, Oh, Ojas!

Ojas keeps all living beings nourished and refreshed.
There can be no life without ojas.

....

CHARAKA SUTRA STHANA, CHAPTER 30, VERSE 9

Remember Iris in the library, pushing eighty and bowling everybody over with her charm and charisma? She had the glow factor big time. It's not necessarily about looking younger, although that is not uncommon. The glow is about living well, feeling confident, and radiating contentment that other people can discern. That way, they won't simply be impressed by how you present yourself: they'll be moved by how they feel in your presence.

The energy we are talking about has a lot to do with the ayurvedic concept of *ojas*. The cosmetic industry has tried for years to somehow bottle this, the quintessence of radiance. Think of how somebody looks and feels after a great vacation or when they are newly in love. This is ojas—"vigor," "fluid of life," "vital sap." That may sound like an expensive serum, but it's not for sale. We generate it ourselves. Signs of abundant ojas include clear, sparkling eyes, a radiant complexion, disease resistance, a pleasant body smell, and bound-out-of-bed energy in the morning.

You are aware at this juncture that the doshas, vata, pitta, and kapha, define and delineate who we are physically. Taking good care of ourselves is meant to keep any one of these from getting out of hand. However, each dosha has a beneficial inner quality, an energy reserve that we could just about always use a little more of. Ojas is this inner aspect of kapha dosha, and it is responsible for the juicy quality that exemplifies youth. It's necessary for strong immunity, good humor, even spiritual fortitude. When ojas is optimal, we're eager to engage in health-promoting and life-enhancing activities. When it isn't, our motivation lags, and so does our energy.

If you are noticing that your skin is drier than usual, you're seeming more susceptible to whatever is going around, your attitude is more than partly cloudy, and you're having trouble with focus, insufficient ojas may be involved. If you are thinking, "Insufficient ojas? This sounds to me like too much vata," go to the head of the class. These are different concepts with overlapping features. When the issue is overabundant vata, we're looking at an excess of its air and ether elements in our system. Low ojas, on the other hand, has to do with lack of energy in the tissues of the body, known in yoga and ayurveda as *dhatus*. But here's the point of connection: imbalanced vata interferes with the good digestion essential for ojas production.

So, let's build up some ojas reserves. Then they will be there to help fight an infection, get the extra oomph for a major project, and start generating some of that "You glow, girl!" appearance. Most whole, plant foods help generate ojas. Among the all-stars are fresh fruits, notably ripe bananas, figs, mangos, and citrus, plus that radiant root, the sweet potato. (You see what's going on. All these foods have some sweetness. Most are soft, or they are after cooking. They're easy to digest, and ill-digested food is the archenemy of ojas and of overall well-being.) Other ojas-uppers include:

- Avocado
- Basmati rice: ayurveda likes basmati (or "fragrant") rice for its digestibility; even though it is not a whole grain, it has a markedly lower glycemic index than white rice and a decent amount of fiber. (Alternatively, you can purchase brown basmati rice, which has not had its outer layer polished off.)
- Blanched almonds: the skins of almonds contain a bitter

substance called tannin that could inhibit the process, but with the skin removed, almonds generate ojas as proficiently as they calm vata dosha.

- Leafy greens and freshly extracted green juices and vegetable juices
- Pink lentils, split mung beans, and tofu
- Sesame seeds and tahini (sesame butter, a traditional ingredient in hummus)
- Spices: cardamom, coriander, and cumin, known as ayurveda's three c's, and saffron, shown in research studies to help with memory loss.
- The rasayana Chyawanprash (see chapter 11, "Spices and Herbs for Rejuvenation") is said to support and protect ojas. According to Gerard C. Buffo, MD, of the Kripalu School of Ayurveda, "It's Ayurveda's standard cure-all, because it decreases the stuff that decreases ojas."

But just as walking comes before running and getting acquainted precedes becoming best friends, boosting ojas happens only after our various dhatus have been nourished. These tissues, according to ayurveda, are *rasa* (plasma—and yes, we've seen that rasa has other meanings; Sanskrit is like English that way), *rakta* (blood), *mamsa* (muscle), *meda* (fat), *asthi* (bones), *majja* (bone marrow), and *shukra* (reproductive tissue). Getting all these thoroughly fed can take some time. This means that going from ho-hum to "Oh, my!" won't happen overnight. Give your body at least a month of plant-based eating with the frequent inclusion of the foods listed above. Then assess: are you feeling more vigor and robustness?

Everything you can do to assist your agni, digestive fire, will power up the process: eating moderate amounts of food in simple combinations, having the main meal at midday, drinking ginger tea and eating ginger pickles, chewing some fennel seeds after meals. An early-to-bed, early-to-rise schedule gives your body the opportunity to appropriate the nutritive and vibrational elements of ojas-building foods. So does regular meditation, sex with someone you trust, good music, and the state of joy. Steady joy is ideal, but surges are good, too, and if drib-bles are all you can conjure at the moment, accept them with gratitude. Exercise is also vital in ojas creation and preservation; so is maintaining an easeful relationship with the exigencies of life. I see this as dancing with what each day presents. You move with the circumstances, observe them without judgment, and add a dip or a twirl when you get the chance.

See yourself as someone brimming with ojas: attractive, sexy, com-fortable in your own skin, radiating good health and good cheer. This is not wishful thinking: it's been shown repeatedly that injured athletes who "practice" mentally while on the sidelines maintain their form and skill level to a far greater degree than those who don't.

We said that ojas is the inner essence of kapha dosha. When it's ample within us, it contributes to the inner essences of vata and pitta doshas too. Pitta's essential essence is *tejas*—inner fire or illumination, the seed of charisma and another source of that sought-after glow; it is also the deep inner power that can fire up our spiritual lives. Vata's subtle soul is *prana*, introduced in the chapter on breathing. Prana, as you'll remember, is life force energy, responsible for our staying alive in these bodies and for maintaining physical, mental, and spiritual har-mony. Because it is ojas that holds the other two essences, however, we can keep things simple: enliven ojas. The rest will take care of itself.

PRACTICES FOR THE PATH

Pack on ojas-enhancing picnic. Make a warm salad of steamed sweet potatoes and baby lentils, spiced with those three c's: cardamom, cori-ander, cumin. Serve on saffron rice. Steep some tulsi or licorice tea. And for dessert make heavenly treat balls by combining equal parts Medjool dates and blanched almonds in a food processor and rolling them, if you like, in some cocoa or carob powder.

Chapter 17

Happy Thoughts

Your thoughts affect your emotions, which affect your
actions. If you can't go from negative to positive,
go from negative to neutral.

....

BARBARA BIZIOU, GLOBAL RITUAL AUTHORITY

Looking on the bright side results in looking brighter, too, at any age. I have seen this all my life in early mentors like Stella and Iris, and contemporaries such as my friend, Dominique, who can find the pot of gold before I have even glimpsed the rainbow. People like these truly *see* the positive. They don't make it up. The rest of us can make it up until we see it. The point of positive seeing, thinking, and living is not simply to make us cheerier people. Our thoughts let our body know how healthy it's supposed to keep us. In this context, the villainous thoughts are called *toxic*, the heroic ones, *tonic*.

Yoga's take on positive thinking is *pratipaksha bhavana*, literally, "opposite sentiment." This is the clever technique of replacing a negative or destructive thought with its antithesis. Ayurvedic doctors recommend this too. Once ingrained, pratipaksha bhavana alerts the brain to negativity the way a fire alarm alerts an engine company. We're then prompted straightaway to replace the thought or impulse that would do us no good. As this becomes a habit, life gets easier. It's not that we're never again in the pathway of Shakespeare's "slings and arrows of outrageous fortune," but we don't make things worse by worrying about where they'll come from next, or replaying the sting of some earlier sling over and over.

Rehearsing messages that no longer serve you (and probably never did) creates tire tracks in your brain: "You never really applied yourself... You're just like your father (or mother)... You should have gone to law school..." It's no wonder we're not abounding in universal optimism. Then age gets involved. A study that looked at 75,000 people from around the world, late teens to 100-plus, determined that optimism increases through mid-adulthood, plateaus from fifty-five to seventy, and then heads south. Interesting. *But it doesn't have to be that way.* We always hear that humans have free will and then we see some statistic and think, "Oh boy, I'm sunk." No, you're not: pull out some free will and call on pratipaksha bhavana, replacing your negative thought with its opposite, whether it's about the age you are or something else.

I love how yoga frames this, because it is saying, "Here's something you can do when your thoughts aren't helping you," rather than, "Shame on you: you had another negative thought." When met with challenging circumstances, perplexing hormones, or assorted slings and arrows, nobody needs to hear "Cheer up: it's not that bad," either from an outside voice or an inner nag. Sometimes things look bad and feel worse. We need to recognize the situation before we can transform it, accept it, or employ some hybrid of the two. In the meantime, it is valid to be with our emotions until they're ready to pass, the way a stalled train will, before long, leave the station. Judgment is so twentieth century.

The twentieth-first has its own challenges. Certainly, creature comforts and technological advances make for an easier life for millions, but even we lucky ones know about and witness images of suffering around the globe every day. This is a lot to process. We must set protective boundaries for ourselves and safeguard our mental health, while at the same time acknowledging that there is a level at which others' suffering is ours, too, because we are connected. All that stuff about being our brother's keeper, and that when the bell tolls, it's as much for us as for the person whose funeral is happening, is more than metaphor.

I have always had good friends and I care about them deeply, but in this age of social media, people I met once on a bus or at an airport are "friends" too. In a way, this is amazing. The sun never sets on our internet empires. It also means that we see really often that someone's mom is seriously ill or their companion animal just passed away. I used to send cards at times like these. I couldn't keep up now, even if I owned controlling interest in Hallmark.

Then there are those closer to us. With age, we start to see people we knew, and public figures we felt we knew, leave this earth. Our friends, people of our vintage, begin to have "old person problems." Good grief, we start to have them ourselves! So, what do we do: affirmations, self-hypnosis, stick our head in the sand? Well, the first two are good. My favorite affirmation hack these days is to hide them within my various computer passwords. Of course, each password has to be different and garnished with numerals and capital letters and punctuation marks, but if you put an affirmation somewhere inside each one, you will be reminded of something you want to learn or accomplish every time some cyber gatekeeper wants to make sure you're really you.

Yoga also has a secret for affirmation effectiveness that is pretty nifty. You couple your denial (not the bad kind, simply a releasing statement of what you want to be rid of) and your affirmation with alternate nostril breathing, nadi shodhana, introduced in chapter 7. You exhale the thing you wish to be rid of, stating that clearly in your mind, e.g., "I breathe out fear." And you inhale what you want to replace it with: "I breathe in courage." This is not a one-time trick, but with sufficient repetition you will impress upon your subconscious that regardless of how things appear, they can be different. Either the circumstance will change or we will. I must admit to favoring the former, but the latter works too, and from a soul perspective, the growth that comes from our changing may be more valuable than getting what we think we want.

PRACTICES FOR THE PATH

Play pratipaksha bhavana. I say "play" because this should be fun. So, let's say that you think to yourself, "God, I did something stupid again." Ding, ding, ding! It's time to play pratipaksha bhavana. Cancel that last thought and replace it with "I am so endearingly human. My imperfections just make me cuter."

Chapter 18

Happy Chakras

The chakras are very intelligent—they are like the software
of the whole computer body.

....

SRI DHARMA MITTRA

I have paid to have my chakras unblocked by colored lights and colored crystals, sound baths and healing hands. I accepted but then regifted to an eight-year-old a chakra coloring book. And I stopped short of investing in the chakra-balancing course in which a youthful Tony Robbins doppelganger would tell me to lift weights, take cold showers, and wear red underwear—and that was just in the free intro session on chakra number one.

Suffice it to say, there is a lot of hype out there around chakras. Let's cut through some of it. The word means "wheel"—chakras are described as "spinning vortexes"—and the "ch" is pronounced as you would in church or chair, not "sh" as in, "Shoot, this is complicated: I just want some glow factor."

The basics are that we have seven primary chakras (see sidebar). Even the fanciest diagnostic machine can't detect these energy swirls because they are not part of the physical body, as hard as that is to grok when we give them names like "heart chakra" and "throat chakra." Some sources place the chakras in the etheric body, others in the astral body. I go with the former because that's where the late Geoffrey Hodson, whom I met and trust, put them, and he saw them. Hodson was a theosophist and clairvoyant who was able to see angels, auras, chakras, and all manner of wondrous things. He described these to an artist and several of his books, some still in print, are so illustrated.

THE SEVEN CHAKRAS

1. *Muladhara,* root (or earth) chakra. Color: red. Relates to: safety and survival. Gems: hematite (bloodstone), garnet. Asanas: mountain, chair pose, child's pose. Affirmation: *I am safe and cared for.* Foundational foods: beets (they're red *and* a root), raspberries, strawberries, red-skinned apples, turnips, cayenne, paprika. Other supports: Get some exercise, engage in a passion project, go outside—digging in the dirt is extra credit.

2. *Svadhisthana,* sacral (or water) chakra. Color: orange. Relates to: sexuality, intimacy, and creativity. Gems: moonstone, orange carnelian, tiger's eye. Asanas: goddess pose, squat. Affirmation: *I am filled with life, artistry, and inspiration.* Foundational foods: orange edibles, such as mango, pumpkin, sweet potatoes, and curry dishes. Other supports: Infuse your indoor air with essential oils including bergamot, sweet orange, or pachouli, or add your favorite to bath water. Also, engage in whatever creative pursuits get your juices going.

3. *Manipura,* solar plexus (or fire) chakra. Color: yellow. Relates to: energy, self-esteem, relationships with others. Gems: lapis lazuli, citrine, yellow tourmaline, amethyst. Asanas: all twists, sun salutation, bow, boat. Affirmation: *I am enough, just the way I am.* Foundational foods: whole grains, pineapple, banana, summer squash, ginger, turmeric. Other supports: Get safe sunlight (a bikini will get some sun to your solar plexus); sit by a fire or other heat source.

4. *Anahata,* heart (or air) chakra. Color: green. Relates to: unconditional love, ability to give and receive love. Gems: lapis lazuli, emerald, rose quartz. Asanas: cobra, cat and cow, bridge pose, half-moon pose. Affirmation: *I am love. I radiate love. I attract love.* Foundational foods: greens and green juices, green tea, cucumber, mint, lime, kiwi. Other supports: Wear green clothing, be around green plants, express gratitude, and mimic the heart's frequency with 341.3 Hz music (it's all over YouTube).

5. *Vishuddha*, throat (or space) chakra. Color: blue. Relates to: communication, truthfulness, direction. Gems: aquamarine, turquoise, lapis lazuli (best worn as a necklace for proximity to the throat). Asanas: all inversions, such as headstand, shoulder stand, legs up the wall; also, fish pose, camel pose, cobra, corpse pose. Affirmation: *I speak clearly, truthfully, powerfully.* Foundational foods: blueberries, blackberries, dragon fruit, plums, purple grapes, coconut water, herbal teas. Other supports: neck stretches and neck massage, bodywork and energy work, journal writing, and speaking in front of people.

6. *Ajna*, third eye (or mind) chakra. Color: indigo. Relates to: focus, intuition, spirituality. Gems: amethyst, black obsidian, clear quartz, black tourmaline. Asanas: child's pose, dolphin pose, warrior 3. Affirmation: *I respect and trust my intuition.* Foundational foods: blueberries, grapes, coffee, cocoa. Other supports: Meditate, optionally visualizing indigo light entering your third eye area with each inhale.

7. *Sahasrara*, crown (or consciousness) chakra. Color: violet (some sources say colorless). Relates to: spiritual enlightenment, unity consciousness. Gems: clear quartz, lapis lazuli, white agate. Asanas: cat and cow, dolphin pose, full forward bend, headstand. Affirmation: *I am divinely guided.* Foundational foods: blueberries, oranges, lychees, and edible violets; also fasting, for those who can do it, or that gentler ayurvedic detox of stewed and spiced apples in the morning, kitchari with your choice of vegetables for the other two meals, plus herbal teas. You can do this up to five days if it's comfortable. Other supports: Keep your environment decluttered, use essential oil of frankincense, meditate (ideally twice a day) and pray ("without ceasing" is good, or whenever you think of it).

David Frawley, MD, author of *Yoga and Ayurveda*, gets down to business when he writes, "The chakras are one of the most popular but misunderstood concepts of yogic thought. Today the chakras are usually presented in a physicalized and distorted manner. Their true nature relates to energy and consciousness, developed through pranayama, mantra, meditation and samadhi." In other words, if we follow the instructions, we will get the results. Colored lights and chakra massage are entertaining, but when it comes to opening our chakras, it has to be an inside job, and it takes as long as it takes.

As Dr. Frawley explains so well in his *Yoga International* article, "Opening the Chakras: New Myths and Old Truths" (I suggest you look this up), some representatives of the New Age and alternative healing worlds imply that chakras are primarily about physical well-being. According to yogic teachings, however, chakras are closed in almost everybody with no apparent pathology as a result. The average person is not incapacitated by chakra stagnation; they are simply not yet on a serious spiritual path and consciously en route to eternal bliss.

Calming the fluctuations of the mind—the goal of yoga, according to Patanjali—will get us there. While this process is not easy, the instructions are simple. First, live a clean life. Yoga's moral precepts and personal disciplines (chapters 24 through 33) and the recommendation of a plant-based diet are all about that. These are valuable prerequisites to making safe and steady progress on the inner journey. Then we move on to concentration, meditation, and connection.

When the kundalini energy, depicted as a pair of intertwined serpents sleeping at the base of the spine, rises through the nadis (energy channels), the chakras open. In his Medium.com article, "Third Eye Opening, Kundalini Awakening, and Enlightenment," Sri Nithra Dridananda writes: "With Kundalini Awakening your bio-memory feels the heat of the consciousness. With Third-Eye opening, your bio-memory feels connected to the conscious presence. And with Enlightenment, your bio-memory becomes One with the conscious presence."

This is way beyond my pay grade, but I occasionally experience times when everybody on the subway looks like an angel. I think these are previews of coming attractions. I'll bet you've had previews too. It is good to enjoy these and not rush anything. Sometimes people are eager to develop psychic powers or hop on an express train to enlightenment. They become involved in very intense breathwork and other activities designed to almost blast open their chakras. It usually doesn't work, and that's good because when it does, actual neurological and psychological damage can occur.

I see the chakras as anchors for self-care, and their descriptors and supports can be viable ways to zero in on an issue. If I need more energy, I look to first chakra remedies: up the exercise; pay more attention to home and hearth-keeping. If it's confidence: third chakra, eat some pineapple, get some sun. If I've been ignoring intuitive signals: sixth chakra, quartz crystals in a little bag, more time in child's pose, schedule a meditation retreat. Everything we're doing to age like yogis supports both our physical well-being and our spiritual growth. If we prioritize the spiritual, the rest takes care of itself, chakras included.

PRACTICES FOR THE PATH

You may have heard it said, "Don't even think about the chakras below the heart: they're so crude." This is chakra snobbery and we don't need it—not in later life anyhow. We're in a curious spot in maturity. We know we are closer to leaving this world than arriving in it, and yet we want to be here in good health for as long as possible. For this reason, we need to stay connected to the energies of security, passion, and confidence that the first three chakras symbolize. So what if they're more about earth than heaven? As one in no hurry to shuffle any mortal coils, I am fine with some earthiness. Maybe those crimson skivvies would have been a good idea after all.

Chapter 19

Beauty Inside and Out

Older people's faces and bodies show so clearly a lifetime
of thinking patterns. How will you look when you are
elderly?... If every day is an awakening, you will never
grow old. You will just keep awakening.

....

LOUISE HAY

Among the many oddities that surround aging in our culture is the notion of "over fifty" as a kind of cut-off, as if one birthday separates youth from age. We would never say "under fifty" to imply that an adult with a job and a mortgage had the same interests and concerns as a second grader. This becomes important as we consider beauty in later life. It's natural at any age to want to appear well to others, but the specter of "looking old" looms largest when we are still relatively young. Later, we would far rather feel good, and if we do, we'll almost invariably look fine. Besides, the visible changes that characterize the passage of time generally come slowly. We get used to them. Being able to look in the mirror at an aging face and say, "I love you, beautiful," helps a lot.

There is also a mystical element at play here. The word "glamour" comes from early eighteenth-century Scotland with the original meaning of "enchantment" or "magic spell." It still works that way. Someone who intrigues you becomes larger than life, whether they are a celebrity or an acquaintance—and it has very little to do with appearance. There's the urban legend about Marilyn Monroe, that she could walk down the street at the height of her fame and go unnoticed until she "turned on Marilyn," claiming the persona. We need to do some of this, too, if we want to age well in a youth-focused culture. We can start by embodying role models, alive and deceased, who have done this. My list includes Iris, Stella, my mom, Maya Angelou, Gloria Swanson, Eleanor Roosevelt, Dolly Parton, and Jane Goodall. Women like these impact us first with their *being*, before any visual first impression.

I once saw Liza Minelli in concert. The curtain went up and there she was—except she wasn't. She was behind a scrim. All we could see was the outline of her body in a wonderful Fosse shape, with one arm stretched stylistically over her head. We had no view of her face and she hadn't sung a note. It took only that suggestion of her presence to get an entire audience out of our seats, all of us screaming like teenagers. That, my friend, was a "glamour" in the traditional sense. We were on our feet screaming because of Liza's talent and tenacity, her life experience and what she had brought to ours, and because she carried both her own legacy and that of her mother.

This is the great big secret to beauty in the—okay, I'll say it—post-fifty decades: *Our lives need to be so exquisite that when someone looks at our face, they see our life.* It doesn't call for the acclaim of the world, just showing up every day, doing our best, allowing for setbacks, and bouncing back from each one, sometimes brilliantly. Every kind word, good deed, selfless act, and creative accomplishment contributes to beauty in later life. We are called upon to rise to our full height, claim our full selves, and remember who we are. We can't expect other people, especially younger ones, to be of much help here. This is on us.

Start with smiling. The muscles smiling involves are also those that lift the lower face, so you will look younger when you do it. In studies, observers register smiling faces as more attractive. When a smile accentuates crow's feet, they go from being wrinkles to crinkles: lines without judgment. And underneath it all, that smile is releasing a slew of feel-good hormones to bolster both mood and immunity.

Frequent smilers apparently even outlive those of more neutral visage. The science as to why this is so remains unclear, but in yogic thought, smiling is very much called for because life on earth is, after all, *maya*, illusion. The illusory nature of things comes in their temporality, but even if all life is a stage, we are expected to turn in an award-worthy performance. Never short on concepts, yoga has another one to lighten things up: *lila*, "God's play." All that is exists because of the creative play of the Creator, and we've been invited to join in the game.

PRACTICES FOR THE PATH

Get to know, for real or by reputation, incredibly cool people who celebrate the age they are. A place to start is with the work of photographer Ari Seth Cohen, founder of the Advanced Style movement (www. advancedstyle.com). It celebrates women in their seventies, eighties, and nineties who make stunning fashion statements. You might want to take a look at the book *Advanced Style*, and the eponymous documentary, blog, and Instagram account.

If fashion isn't your thing, find mature role models in your areas of interest. This is not about imitating what others do—that's for middle school, not middle age and later. Case in point: I don't copy-cat what the Advanced Style ladies wear, both because I know how I like to dress, and I am committed to a fully vegan wardrobe. But the women Cohen photographs have carved a template for sartorial self-expression in later life, inspiring those who discover them to treat the sidewalk as a runway: Models Sought. All Ages.

Chapter 20

Skin, Hair, and Ayurveda

*It is limiting and ultimately detrimental to think of
beauty as something dependent upon the shape and
features of our anatomy.*

....

PRATIMA RAICHUR, MATRIARCH OF AYURVEDIC SKIN CARE

When we think of aging, we think of skin and hair because they are obvious. Some of the problems we have with skin are straight-forward: discoloration, blotchiness, and lines that result from long-term sun exposure. Other skin complaints of the post-youth era, however, have to do with its supporting structures. Production of collagen, a protein that keeps our skin from sagging, starts to decrease before we turn thirty. That lovely layer of fat we seldom appreciate when we're young diminishes (thanks, vata), and the fully calcified bones that give our facial skin its foundation can start to erode.

The upshot: we're challenged to care of our skin and its support systems for the long haul. Sun protection and not smoking pay massive dermal dividends. Hydration matters, inside and out. Even sleeping on our backs instead of our sides, saving cheeks from the nightly tug of a pillow, is a good habit to adopt. And we need to take care of our dominant dosha as it comes through in our skin. Consider your own prakriti, the result of the dosha quiz you took, and also your stage of life and what is showing up on your very own face.

- Kapha is prominent in childhood when skin is usually flawless.

Even in old age, those with substantial kapha influence tend to have beautiful complexions. Kapha cheeks stay round and plump, and this dosha ages well. Kapha folks may have to deal with oily skin and enlarged pores, and perhaps a tendency toward fluid retention and puffy eyes in the morning; cucumber slices and cooled black tea bags on eyelids can lessen this.

- Too much fiery pitta, higher in all of us from puberty through middle age, can lead to breakouts, redness, and broken capillaries. Avoid hot spices, piping hot drinks, and alcohol. Use cool compresses on your face if you've overheated. Aloe vera on the skin, either commercial or from the plant itself, is a great soother.

- In later life when vata increases, we are likely to be dealing with thinner, drier skin, and a proclivity to lines and wrinkles. Oil counteracts vata, so look for products that are oily, slippery, and rich. Because vata is systemic, the warm oil massage that you're doing some mornings adds to your youthful appearance, not just because you're applying oil to your face but because the process calms vata overall. Sipping warm water and herbal teas throughout the day and eating a high-water-content diet— fruits, veggies, low-sodium soups, low-sugar juices—provides moisture from within. Ingested oils, notably those in whole foods—nuts, seeds, avocado—also play a role in saving face.

All the suggestions in the sidebar, here, are on the natural side. Even so, a good dermatologist can do amazing things. Seeing one for elective reasons falls under maintenance. If you are at the higher end of the maintenance scale, claim it if you can, and if you're a high maintainer still in the workforce, *save more money*. It's expensive to be old if you want to take care of cosmetic concerns and avail yourself of alternative therapeutics which Medicare and backup plans almost never cover.

SKIN CARE FOR YOGIS OF A CERTAIN AGE

Lifestyle
- Sun protection, no midday sun. SPF 30 or higher daily, even

indoors (UVA, as in aging, rays come through glass); reapply natural barrier sunscreen every two to four hours. Sunglasses, brimmed hats, and gloves. No alcohol, nothing through a straw. Pacify vata with comforting foods, warmth, ample sleep, peace and quiet. Stress management (the stress hormone cortisol inhibits collagen production). Body care services: oil massage and *shirodara* (a stream of warm sesame oil caressing the third eye area, available at ayurvedic clinics and spas). Annual dermatologist checkup for skin cancer screening and, if you're interested, a cosmetic consult. *Panchakarma*, "five treatments," healing and detoxification protocol, annually if possible, at an ayurvedic clinic, retreat center, or spa.

Diet

- Oranges, strawberries, peppers, and amla (Indian gooseberry, available frozen and powdered) contain vitamin C, involved in collagen synthesis.

- Pumpkin seeds, hemp seeds, cashews, quinoa, and dark chocolate provide zinc, which aids in collagen production.

- Mulberries, black currants, cherries, raspberries, pomegranate, red cabbage, purple cauliflower, and purple sweet potato are rich in anthocyanins, antioxidants that protect against UV rays, as well as against inflammation and certain carcinogens.

- Carrots, pumpkin, sweet potato, winter squash, apricots, cantaloupe, mangoes, and citrus have carotenoids, which protect skin from UV radiation, pollution, and smoke; and when Caucasian subjects who had consumed these freely were compared to others who hadn't, the carrot eaters were judged sexier by a panel of strangers.

- Legumes, i.e., black beans, pinto beans, soybeans, and soy products aid in the production of elastin, which gives skin its ability to stretch and return to its proper shape; beans also contain antioxidants that protect the skin from free radical damage.

- Low-salt soups, fresh fruits, and leafy greens provide hydration, and avocado, nuts, seeds, and extra virgin olive oil provide lubrication. Limit dehydrating substances: caffeine, alcohol, salty snacks, added sugar, animal protein.
- Cinnamon, ginger, turmeric, cloves, and all other spices except salt are antioxidant power players. Spice up everything. Using spice blends, such as pumpkin pie spice, Italian seasoning, herbes de Provence, garam masala, and curry powder makes it easier to get an array of these.

Herbs: Tulsi, amla, ashwagandha

Asanas: Fish, camel, triangle, and all inversions

Care routine: This comes from Melanie A. Sachs, author of *Ayurvedic Beauty Care: Ageless Techniques to Evoke Natural Beauty*:

1. Bathe your face thoroughly with warm water. "Dead skin cells will soak up the water like little sponges and plump up, which makes them easy to remove."

2. Make an *ubtan* (ayurvedic cleansing powder) with 2 tablespoons of oat flour and 1 tablespoon of water. Bend over the sink, dip your second, third, and fourth fingertips into the ubtan, and gently press the paste onto your face. This removes the dead skin cells without stripping the skin of its natural oils.

3. Put some plain water or rose water in a spray bottle and spritz the face a few times to moisten the skin. While the face is still wet, apply a thin coating of jojoba oil to seal in the moisture. (Jojoba oil is closest to the skin's sebum; it is highly unlikely to cause irritation.)

And then there's hair. My mom was a cosmetologist, so I grew up in beauty shops. As perplexing to the six-year-old me as the headlines in *Photoplay* and *True Confessions* was an even bigger mystery: why the gramma-aged ladies almost all had the same hairdo—short, curly, with bangs. I have since learned that they had the same hairstyle because they had the same hair. Now I have it too. Left to its own devices, third act hair is apt to be as dry as June in Las Vegas. Lack of melanin means that gray or white hair can turn frizzy and coarse, whether virgin or colored. Not only that: as we get older, our hair follicles themselves change, going from round to squarish. If your hair feels rough or frizzy, take heart: you're dealing with square hair. Who knew?

So, we assess. This is personal (it's growing out of your head, for heaven's sake), and racial and ethnic specifics also need to be considered when we are caring for our coifs. In general, kapha dosha is behind thick, healthy hair, *and* we would all do well to calm the drying influences of excess vata. Hair loss, known in modern science as hereditary and hormonal, is linked in ayurveda to overabundant pitta. The theory is that pitta's heat weakens hair follicles, and this often starts in our forties when pitta is at its zenith.

It may be daunting to feel that you must look out for pitta to keep your hair full and look out for vata to keep it shiny, so simplify by focusing more on vata during vata season (fall through early winter) and more on pitta during the summer. It's intuitive, because we all want more hot soup and early nights (good for vata) when the weather is colder, and more juicy fruits and water aerobics (good for pitta) when it's hot.

If thinning hair is a concern, it is one I share with you. It can be tough on the self-esteem, despite affirming "I am not my body, I am not my body." The basics are to protect hair from sunlight, drink plenty of water, and keep up with meditation and other stress-management techniques. Be sure your diet is adequate in protein, iron, zinc, and B-complex vitamins.

Do scalp massage as often as you can when you perform abhyanga, and perhaps use cooling coconut oil or aloe vera gel instead of sesame oil, at least for your head. There is also a product from India, available online, called Indulekha Bringha Hair Oil, that a lot of people swear by. The active ingredient is an herb called *bringha*, long recommended in ayurvedic medicine to counteract hair loss. A sub-specialty beneath the ayurvedic umbrella is *marma therapy*, in which certain points are massaged or stimulated, similar to what you may have experienced in trigger point massage or acupressure. Some of these marmas, "vulnerable points," on the head are related to hair growth and restoration. Several YouTubers offer instruction; I like the channel @sushmitasdiaries.

Inversion postures such as headstand, unless otherwise contraindicated (see chapter 6), are also said to help with hair growth. And even though shedding hair can be sufficiently depressing to make you want to stop brushing, try to get past that and do at least a little daily brushing; the scalp stimulation should help in the long run.

Western science has made meaningful strides around hair loss. Some of these are quite natural, i.e., topically applied rosemary oil, in one study rivaling minoxidil (Rogaine), the first FDA-approved hair restoration treatment. If you need more backup, visit a dermatologist, trichologist, or a reputable hair restoration clinic. There are topical and oral medications, laser light devices, and treatments such as PRP (platelet-rich plasma, spun down from your own blood and injected into the scalp) that appear to regrow hair for some people. In the meantime, a hairdresser with an interest in mature or thinning hair can do more than you might think with the right cut and style.

The bottom line on the cosmetic aspects of growing older is that change happens. Hairs can start to sprout from your chin around the same time that eyebrow hairs stop growing (applying castor oil nightly can help with the eyebrows). The same woman can have a face that looks fifty and hands that look seventy. Gravity isn't lifting anything up. Hard-built muscles may be covered with crêpey skin.

These are facts. But there's also Truth. Capital T. That Truth is that you are eternal, ageless, timeless, and just as you're supposed to be. If something about any aspect of your exterior falls short of somebody's notion of ideal—even *your* notion of ideal—you've simply got to rock it. Be who you are and how you are at this moment. Approve of yourself. Appreciate yourself. Show up confident with no apologies. Now, that's beautiful.

PRACTICES FOR THE PATH

Celebrate silver. I still get my hair colored (with Aveda, cruelty free and less toxic than conventional brands), but by the time you read this book, with my brown-haired picture on the cover, I may have given it up. I am entranced by others' natural tresses—as well as those bohemian beauties who streak their silver with purple or some other flamboyant hue. You can follow pro-natural-color influencers on social media and check out books such as *Gray Hair Adventure: Things I Learned About Life When I Stopped Dyeing My Hair*, by Susan Paget, and *Silver Hair: Say Goodbye to the Dye and Let Your Natural Light Shine*, by Lorraine Massey and Michele Bender.

Part Six

In Search of Sattva

Chapter 21

Googling the Gunas

Guna means strand: in the Gita the gunas are described as the very fabric of existence, the veil that hides unity in a covering of diversity.

....

VYASA, COMPILER OF THE MAHABHARATA

We can all remember past yearnings—to be popular in school, get into a particular college, land the right job, find the perfect partner. A perk of spiritual practice is to free us from yearnings, except for the overarching longing for *moksha*, liberation. Recognizing how difficult it is to turn from tangible desires, yoga offers something that won't take us all the way to the goal of Self-realization but will, like one of those moving walkways at the airport, get us quite a bit closer. This is the cultivation of *sattva*, the mode of purity and balance, one of those three veils that Vyasa tells us in the epigraph shrouds oneness with multiplicity.

All physical life and activity can be categorized under one of three *gunas* or fundamental forces, essential aspects of nature, given the names *tamas, rajas,* and *sattva*. Confusion alert: we've talked quite a bit about the three doshas and their role in our physical and psychological lives. The gunas are something different. Are gunas and doshas related? Yes, because this is yoga and everything is related. But you don't have to worry about that here. Just open some fresh mental circuitry and welcome in a new idea: the three gunas. For life on earth to proceed, each of them is necessary.

Tamas is the energy of non-energy—inertia, decay. While tamas covers such unsavory areas as sloth and crime, the great balm of sleep is also a tamasic process; so is what happens in a compost bin. Rajas is energy on steroids—it's action, innovation, even aggression. Rajasic energy builds families and civilizations, although rage and out-of-control passions are rajasic too. Sattva is balance—beauty, purity, peace. Like Mary Poppins and your dog, sattva is practically perfect.

Healing is sattvic. So is spiritual growth. Natural and esthetic beauty, valor and love, divine connection through any religion or no religion—file all these under sattva. Art, music, poetry, drama—creativity of all kinds, as well as appreciation of others' creativity—are divine in origin and sattvic in nature. So are kindness and charity, the ways we bring heaven to earth. Even small courtesies count: "Thank you." "My pleasure." A gift for the host. A note in the lunchbox.

Do you garden? You make sattvic space. Are you a birdwatcher or nature photographer? You have a sattvic hobby. Do you sew or craft? That's sattva with a needle and a glue gun. Do you sing in a choir or have tickets for chamber music next weekend? Harmonic sattva. Do you read to a blind person or volunteer at a shelter? Sattva of the heart. Sattva is not difficult to recognize or cultivate. We need only to live in a higher-vibe state and be consistent about it. Just as showing up for classes doesn't guarantee graduation, living a sattvic life does not guarantee enlightenment, but it gets you in the ballpark, or the ballpark parking lot.

A delicious way to increase the sattvic element in your body and your life is to eat sattvic foods. "When we eat sattvic food, it gives us inner clarity, determination and peace," Om Swami writes in *The Wellness Sense*. "Rajasic food fuels our passions, and tamasic food creates aggression and restlessness." If you're feeling overloaded with dietary advice, I get it. First, yoga says our food should be nonviolent and natural. We expect it to build our health and our ojas and keep our doshas in balance. And now it's got a guna?

It is okay. The wonderful thing about yoga's nutritional suggestions is that the same foods show up over and over as either discouraged or recommended. Sometimes you will see a food labeled tamasic on one list and rajasic on another. Simplify by making sattvic choices most of the time.

- *Tamasic foods are said to deplete prana, dull the mind, cause lethargy and lack of motivation, and promote negative emotions, even depression. Yogis generally avoid these altogether.* Examples: meat, fish, eggs, leftovers (the longer they are left, the more tamasic they get), highly processed foods, alcohol.
- *Rajasic foods are stimulating; eating too much of them may promote covetousness and belligerence, and interfere with the delicate body/mind connection; yogis consume these in moderate amounts, if at all.* Examples: caffeine, refined sugar, vinegar, fried food, and an excess of salt or hot spices, such as peppers and chiles. (Onion and garlic are also rajasic, although esteemed by modern nutritional science.)
- *Sattvic foods are nourishing to body and soul.* Vegetables, fruits, whole or sprouted grains, legumes, nuts, seeds, and most spices, including basil, cinnamon, coriander, fennel, ginger, saffron, and turmeric are sattvic. Traditional listings include dairy, but I agree with points made by Ankur Bhatia in his online article, "What About Milk? What About Nutrition? What About Tradition?" He writes, "Ayurveda says that milk is *sattvic* in its properties. But we can say that it gets *tamasic* when we factor in how animals are treated to extract the milk, milk processing, form of consumption and the quantity in which it is consumed."

This is in keeping with the teaching that what is done to a food—and, in this case, what is done to the being who produced the food—can alter its guna. For example, a sattvic sweet potato would become rajasic if turned into sweet potato fries; if you kept those fries in the fridge a few days and reheated them, they would wind up tamasic.

When the foods you choose are freshly picked, purchased, and prepared, and when they taste really, really good, you can feel an energetic shift. I had an experience with this once in Sedona, a place known to be spiritual and cosmic, but I was not having a good time. My hotel was at the edge of town and not the good edge. There was a lot of traffic and the January weather was much colder than I'd expected of Arizona. Driving on the main thoroughfare, I noticed to my right a restaurant called ChocolaTree. Some signage indicated that the fare was plant-based, so I pulled in.

The parking spots bore positive quotations, a good start. Once inside, I ordered soup and an entrée. When I tasted the soup—carrot ginger or butternut squash, I don't know; it was orange—the tension of the trip, the cold I wasn't dressed for, and my regret at letting a third-party website choose my hotel evaporated. My first thought was: *What's in this? It can't be legal.* But warmth and freshness and well-chosen spices don't break any laws. In fact, they uphold some: the laws of nature. I knew as a yoga student that sattvic foods increase calmness, clarity, and joy, but I never expected to experience all this so fully—or so quickly. Sattvic soup saved the day.

PRACTICES FOR THE PATH

Become a sattva sleuth. Observe your life to see where sattva shows up. Notice the sattvic foods in your kitchen: vegetables, fruits, seeds, sprouts, greens, grains, and the rest. Look for sattvic activities on your calendar: yoga class, poetry night, your volunteer gig. Take the time to watch a sunset, write your memoir or a thank you note, or walk somewhere you'd have otherwise driven, simply because it is a beautiful day and you want to be out in it, soaking up sattva and feeling terrific. Refrain from multi-tasking, second-guessing, jumping to conclusions, and making do when you know that life has something better for you—something simpler, more peaceful, more sattvic, more you.

Chapter 22

Get Comfy

But Piglet is so small that he slips into a pocket, where it is very comfortable to feel him when you are not quite sure whether twice seven is twelve or twenty-two.

....

A.A. MILNE, *WINNIE-THE-POOH*

When you've had enough with new information and appropriating concepts that seem to lead to another and another and another, it can be priceless to pause and pull together what you've gleaned from your reading, listening, contemplating, and intuiting. When you do that, you can breathe life into all the ideation and fabricate something exquisite for yourself: a nice, comfy life.

In ayurveda, comfort is a requisite of balance for striving pitta, generous kapha, and sensitive vata. Just as babies learn over time to self-soothe, we can learn to self-comfort. We may have been told all our lives that seeking comfort was selfish and lazy. No. That would be overwork, overworry, overcaring, then feeling awful about it and attempting to compensate with late nights and tortilla chips.

You are your own amazing and unique creation, and I'm sure you have ways to comfort yourself that wouldn't seem very comforting to me—camping, maybe. To each their own. To follow are some suggested tidings of comfort and joy, ayurvedically inspired and sanctioned:

- Blankets feel like God's gift to morning, even though we've sworn off the snooze button and are discovering the awe of being up by 6 a.m. But you can set your clock fifteen minutes early, stay snuggled under those comforting comforters, and listen to morning affirmations. That's a quarter-hour more duvet time *and* an upgraded attitude for your day. Thanks to YouTube, we can still hear from Louise Hay and Dr. Wayne Dyer, even though they're no longer in physical life.

- A warm-to-almost-hot bath is the ultimate in comfort, especially for an I-don't-want-to-be-frazzled-but-sometimes-I-am vata (or vata-imbalanced) person. A bath is fine with no accessorizing, but it's easy to put those little battery-powered tea lights around the bathroom, add a couple of drops of lavender oil to a tablespoon or sesame or olive oil and drizzle that into the tub, and maybe play an audiobook. I love listening to Eknath Easwaran's *The Bhagavad Gita for Daily Living*. There is so much meaning in the Gita, the Song of God, the Indian scripture that has long illuminated and comforted people of many faiths around the world. And Easwaran's interpretations of it are so insightful, this recording stays new through countless listens (and countless baths).

- Keep your head warm. If you are largely vata or kapha, you're probably cold a lot and not one to take to winter winds, a superfluous ceiling fan, or an assertive A/C. I always wear a stretchy cap or ear-covering headband when I'm outside or in drafty places. A scarf around the neck calms vata too.

- Keep your feet warm. When you're out in shoes and socks, your feet can get cold because they have become moist. Carry extra socks and change at midday. It will make you feel better than you think something this simple could. If you experience seriously cold toes, get your thyroid checked, but if that's okay, it could be vata imbalance. I generally don't recommend anything disposable, but these are such a godsend for the cold-footed, I must share: skiers' toe warmers. You stick them to the bottom of your socks and then put your shoes on. They're good for about six hours.

- Talk to yourself. "We've got this." "Come on, you've slayed dragons bigger than this one before breakfast." "Miracles happen every day, and this is a day." We have to be our own best friend. In probably my favorite NDE (near-death experience) book, *Dying to Be Me*, Anita Moorjani speaks repeatedly of her time in the hereafter being told "things that pertain to me," "information relevant to my life"—not in a self-centered way but in a way that points to the incredible importance of each one of us, our own life experience, our own circle of loved ones, and our particular sphere of influence.

- Take pleasure in a hot drink. Once a week I treat myself to a chai latté at a coffee place. I can trace the pathway of that barista-blessed beverage down my gullet, warming and soothing and comforting the heck out of me. I am convinced that the hormonal response to all that pleasure more than makes up for the sugar I'm consuming, but plain tea, herbal tea, or hot almond milk with spices can take the edge off and keep you straight-edge too. Whatever your beverage of choice, sip. Delight. Enjoy.

- "In quietness and confidence shall be your strength." My governess-guru, Dede, loved that line from Isaiah and said it all the time. To this day, when I walk into a church or a library and hear the quiet, I also hear her reciting, "In quietness and confidence shall be your strength." Quiet is so valuable. A lot of older folks have tinnitus, ringing of the ear. I've had it for years—bad idea to fly with an ear infection—so the closest I get to silence is white noise coming through a headset or tinnitus masker, but even that is such an upgrade from a noisy city in a noisy century. Maybe you deal with a clamorous job or rambunctious neighbors or a hearing-impaired spouse who cranks up the TV. Find some quiet. It will calm your vata and give you comfort.

- Be sure you're being touched. Statistically, older adults get less touch than any other age group, leading to clinical determinations like "tactile hunger" and "touch starvation." Don't be a statistic. If you have a truelove, you are blessed beyond measure:

cuddle! If you have grandchildren, OMG: cuddle before they become too teenish to get that close. And if you have a companion animal, snuggle up. If you can avail yourself of some sort of bodywork, do that too.

You have probably already realized that as you nurture your inner life, your spiritual practices themselves become comforting. This is the comfort/sattva connection. Simply sitting in your freshly cleaned—no chemicals—room with an hour set aside to perform asanas, meditate, read, journal, or talk with a friend you admire can be such a precious time. This is when comfort and contentment and gratitude get all mixed and blended, and you think that maybe you're the luckiest person on earth.

PRACTICES FOR THE PATH

Where can you add more comfort to your life? Can you do something seriously comforting within the next twenty-four hours?

Chapter 23

The People Who Have Your Back

*However, community is first of all a quality of the heart. It
grows from the spiritual knowledge that we are alive not
for ourselves but for one another.*

....

HENRI J.M. NOUWEN

You may have read about cave-dwelling yogis in the Himalayas who
rarely see other humans and spend all their time in transcendent
ecstasy. Cool. The rest of us need a little spiritual circle, a group of people
who are also seeking to grow. They keep us motivated. They remind us
that we aren't weird or out of touch; we are precisely where we are supposed to be, even if a sibling or a coworker doesn't know what to make
of us.

The blue zones evidence and research studies on longevity concur
that closeness and contact extend lifespans and healthspans. All healthy
closeness is good. Family is family, and they are ours. Friends we've had
forever are family in every way except DNA. It is a cliché that elders
harp on health and family, but there comes a time when things get very
clear. You need to be present and functional (that's the health piece), and
you need to have loving connections because, as Emily Dickinson put it,
"That Love is all there is/ Is all we know of Love."

In the upcoming chapter on truth, you'll find a prayer that begins,
"Lead us from the unreal to the real." That refers to the ultimate reality,
coming to know the Divine as all and everything. But while we live
on earth, some things are more real than others. Love is definitely up

there. When we are young, other things—like winning, achieving, beating somebody else out for the job or the accolade—seem as real as can be and very important. After many decades of life experience, however, people usually come to see that health means the world as long as we're in the world, and love means more—in this world and beyond it. Therefore, it is extra special if some of the people you love the most are part of your little spiritual circle. If, however, your kith and kin have no interest in joining you in this, love them to the tenth power of infinity anyway. And find your spiritual family.

I have long appreciated the company of just about anybody who has a spiritual life. We may not agree on theological precepts, but we share the conviction that life itself has a purpose and individual lives do too. Sometimes there is a friend or relative who insists that they have the only way for everybody to have a spiritual life, and yours isn't the right one. Such a person can certainly be in your life but not part of your little spiritual circle. This is reserved for people who can unabashedly celebrate your spiritual journey, wherever it takes you. In Buddhism, they call a tight-knit group of seekers like this a *sangha*. It is heartwarming to read what people like revered writer Naomi Wolf have to say about being part of one. For most of us, it needn't be that formal. Maybe it's not even a group per se, but a constellation of people who care about you from your soul on out, and you care right back.

PRACTICES FOR THE PATH

Establish a little spiritual circle. To the belief that age and culture are formidable barriers destined to cut people off from one another, your spiritual circle says "Rubbish!" You can start with one other person. If your circle takes off, stop adding members just before the group gets to the verge of outgrowing itself.

The Yamas: Moral Precepts

Chapter 24

Ahimsa: Compassion in Action

Wisdom is knowing we are all One. Love is what it feels like and compassion is what it acts like.

....

ETHAN WALKER III, AUTHOR OF *DEATH OF THE EGO*

Nowadays you can find a yoga class at your gym or on your laptop. All you have to do to take part is pay up and show up—sometimes even the paying is optional. Traditionally, mastery of the *yamas*, the moral precepts covered in this section, and the *niyamas*, personal disciplines to be explored in Part Eight, came first. If you, like most students of yoga in our era, started your exploration with asana, you entered through a helpful and healing door. Just be sure you pick up the prerequisites.

The yamas deal with how we relate to others (even though at the core of the teaching, there really are no "others"). First and foremost is ahimsa, introduced in chapter 8 when I told you Professor Rynn Berry's parable about doing whatever it might take to save that deer from the hunter. While its direct translation is "non-killing" or "non-injury," ahimsa is so much more. One of my early mentors, H. Jay Dinshah, called it "dynamic harmlessness." He said that if someone fell on a city sidewalk and you walked past thinking, "Not my problem; I didn't trip the guy," you might squeak by on the letter of the ahimsa law but woefully miss its spirit.

Ahimsa means that we are to cause as little harm to our fellow beings as possible *and* do the most good we can. Not only that: it admonishes us to speak kind words and even to think kind thoughts. Don't chastise yourself about thoughts; they have a way of popping up unbidden. Nevertheless, just as you are attempting to replace negative notions about yourself with positive ones, do your best to move up a notch any thoughts that are resentful, envious, or demeaning toward others. We tell the people we care about that we wish them well. Ahimsa challenges us to wish everybody well.

SOME WAYS TO EXPRESS AHIMSA

- *Be kind and gentle to yourself.* Ahimsa is about how we treat others, but it starts close to home. Think well of yourself and speak kindly to yourself. Be kind to your body with healthy food and nontoxic products (the Environmental Working Group maintains an up-to-date list of the cleanest body care brands at www.ewg.org/skindeep/). Refrain from overwork if you can, and if you can't—because you're a caregiver or raising grandchildren or holding down two jobs when you thought you'd be retired—find ways to get needed recuperation time. It's not indulgent; it's essential.

- *Learn about nonviolent communication* (www.cnvc.org), a way of expressing ourselves based on the concept of Universal Human Needs. We are more alike than different and we communicate most effectively when empathy underlies our words.

- *Exemplify ahimsa online.* In the anonymity of the internet, people feel justified in making comments that range from unnecessary to horrifying. Don't be one of them. Bill Wilson, cofounder of Alcoholics Anonymous, put it superbly: "Nothing pays off like restraint of tongue and pen." That also goes for clicking "post" or "send."

- *Separate the believer from their beliefs.* We all have opinions and ways of seeing issues. If we had the identical life experiences as someone whose views on politics or something else are opposite ours, we would almost certainly hold the same opinions they do. Besides, a loved one with a position we find absurd is still someone we love. You and I have lived long enough to know that opinions come and go; love can last forever if we give it a chance.

- *Widen your circle.* In a letter written in 1950, Albert Einstein states that our belief in separateness is "a kind of optical delusion of consciousness," and that "Our task must be to free ourselves from this prison by widening our circles of compassion to embrace all living creatures and the whole of nature in its beauty." As our circles widen, those of all humanity do too. When I was in school, we spoke of "mankind." That evolved to "humankind." When we get to "livingkind," we'll have come a long way indeed.

This first yama asks only that we face any situation as nonviolently as is possible and reasonable. This isn't passivity: the Bhagavad Gita is set on a battlefield, a metaphor for the battle of life, and the gist of the Gita is Krishna's urging Arjuna to do his duty as a soldier. Most of us, thank goodness, are not in a war zone today, but the challenge is similar: to show up with a pure heart and valiant intentions. There is even an asana called peaceful warrior, *viparita virabhadrasana.* Sometimes called reverse warrior, this is a chest opener that calms and balances the nervous system. I find it a powerful reminder that the term "peaceful warrior" doesn't have to be an oxymoron.

We can acknowledge ahimsa when confronted with a careless driver, an inflexible bureaucrat, or a belligerent know-it-all on social media simply by acting on the Golden Rule. Ahimsa is hardwired into the timeless teaching of treating others as we wish to be treated, and it won't steer you wrong. As you go deeper into the principle of ahimsa, you'll come to see that everything you have and do and buy and engage in has a history. Even something as prosaic as an item on a menu, shoes in a shop window, or your regular brand of shampoo has a backstory that involved kindness or cruelty, life or death. You can choose which histories to sanction and which industries and companies to support. Before long, you will find yourself at the center of a grand adventure not dependent on age or position. This is the gift of ahimsa: peace and power and purpose, all wrapped up in a box with your name on it.

PRACTICES FOR THE PATH

Take steps in a veganward direction. AI predicts that, due to the huge toll animal agriculture takes on the planet, the world will be functionally vegan by 2075. Why not be an early adapter? There is no simpler, more direct way to practice ahimsa. In refraining from animal products, you—you alone, one person—end the suffering and slaughter of an estimated 200 animals per year. You shrink your carbon footprint up to sixty percent. You play a part in alleviating world hunger by freeing up foodstuffs to feed people directly, instead of wastefully cycling them through the bodies of doomed animals. You honor your arteries and, in that remarkable way that what goes around comes around, you increase your joy. Here are some assists:

- Start with a starter guide—they're free. Download the African American Vegan Starter Guide at www.byanygreensnecessary.com/starter guide; or order the Peta Vegan Starter Kit (in print—they'll mail it) from www.peta.org/living/food/free-vegan-starter-kit/.
- Do an immersion for info and support. If a new year is coming, be part of Veganuary (www.veganuary.com) and join with thousands across the globe in a supported trial of living vegan for the month of January. Or online any time, jump on a 21-Day Vegan Kickstart from Physicians Committee for Responsible Medicine—www.pcrm.org/vegankickstart, or get the app.
- Get to know the beings you're saving by visiting a sanctuary for formerly farmed animals. A robust (but not exhaustive) global list of such sanctuaries can be found at https://vegan.com/blog/sanctuaries/.
- If you travel and want to find suitable food around the world, check out Happy Cow: www.happycow.com or the Happy Cow app.
- For customized guidance, consider working for a time with a vegan lifestyle coach and educator; I can vouch for the ones

certified through Main Street Vegan Academy, a program I founded. If you have specific nutritional challenges and would like to consult with a registered dietitian who understands plant-based eating, find one through the Vegetarian Nutrition Practice Group of the Academy of Nutrition and Dietetics (www.vndpg.org/home).

Chapter 25

Satya: Speak Truth, Live Truth

The entire world is wandering about in search of the truth (satya). The absolute Self which has already become illuminated within. . .is the eternal truth, and it is this that needs to be sought.

....

PARAM PUJYA DADA BHAGWAN

Satya means truth, essential and unembroidered. When Mahatma Gandhi set about to do the impossible, free his country from British colonial rule, he called his movement *satyagraha*, "truth force." This implies that truthfulness goes far beyond not telling lies: it carries power. The root word *Sat* means not only "truth" but Universal Spirit, Brahman, Source, First Cause. This concept shows up other places too. In John 4:16-17, Jesus conflates truth with the Holy Ghost, part of the trinitarian nature of God in Christianity: "the Father will give you another Counselor, to be with you forever, even the Spirit of truth." And one explanation of the healings of Jesus is that he was so imbued in truth that any words he spoke would manifest. If he said, "Take up your bed and walk," that had to happen, prognosis notwithstanding.

In the last century, we have seen satyagraha at work not only in Gandhi's accomplishments but in the tactics of one of his most distinguished proponents, Martin Luther King, Jr. We see it also in addiction recovery. Nearly a century ago, when it was universally believed that the only outcome of alcoholism was institutionalization or death, the writers of *Alcoholics Anonymous* stated, "Rarely have we seen a person fail who has thoroughly followed our path. Those who do not recover are. . .usually men and women who are constitutionally incapable of being honest with themselves."

By speaking, facing, and living the truth, we greatly increase our chances for coming to know it and experience its power in our lives. Do note that satya does not call for the kind of brutal honesty that unnecessarily hurts people. Ahimsa, nonviolence—including nonviolent communication—always comes first.

Do you remember the first lie you ever told? I do. I was in kindergarten, and Dede, my "adopted grandmother," asked what I'd done at school that day. The usual "We sang and colored and drank juice and took a nap" seemed so banal that with nary a moment's forethought, I blurted out, "We rode horses."

As soon as I said it, a pall fell over me. I had lost my innocence. I was still a child in age and stature, but I was now somehow adulterated. And I quickly learned that lying demands more lies, as Dede wanted to know where the horses were kept and the name of my trusty steed. I burst into tears, sobbing, "There were no horses. I just wish there were horses." True to her characteristic refusal to become perturbed, Dede said, "Sometimes we want our wishes to have already happened. It's just important to know the difference between what really happened and what you want for later." That was all very nice, but I'd lost my innocence just the same. And I believe we lose it again every time we attempt to rewrite reality to make ourselves look better or our lives seem easier.

In addition to speaking the truth, however, satya asks that we accept the truth and live accordingly. For example, we need to accept the age we are. That doesn't mean that we should have to retire because somebody says it's time, or dress in some dour and dowdy fashion, or buy into random limitations imposed by society. It does mean that we need to tend to the responsibilities of someone our age—screenings and checkups, a retirement account and a living will. If anyone likes thinking about this stuff, it's nobody I know. It is just necessary. And reasonable. And honest.

Finally, satya asks that we get in touch with our personal truth, living as fully as possible from our authentic nature, even if we come under pressure to modify or conform. We can excavate some of our authenticity by asking ourselves, "What do *I* feel? What do *I* believe? What makes sense *to me*? What is important *to me*?" You can be fully honest only by knowing what you really think and acting accordingly.

Now, perhaps more than ever before, we are aware of ideas and interpretations of reality that are not our own. In addition to the influences of tradition, family, friends, and authority figures, we're constantly fed information by advertisers, media, and—heaven forbid!—bots. Much of what we think we know is reflected truth—or reflected falsehood. The more we engage in the yogic art of *self*-reflection (see chapter 32), the more we'll be able to differentiate between what resonates deeply with us and what is more of a working hypothesis that we might do well to amend or discard.

PRACTICES FOR THE PATH

Say a prayer to know the truth. Any sincere ask should work, but the Pavamana Mantra from the Brihadaranyaka Upanishad is beautiful as both a Sanskrit chant and an invocation in English. You may have heard it in a yoga class and there are dozens of recordings online. It goes as follows; the one untranslated word, Om, etiologically kin to "amen" and "ameen," is said to be the primordial sound that sparked creation and sustains it:

> Om, Asato ma sadgamaya
> Tamaso ma jyotirgamaya
> Mrityorma amritam gamaya
> Om, shanti, shanti, shanti!

And in translation:

> Om, Lead me from the unreal to the real.
> Lead me from darkness to the light.
> Lead me from the fear of death to the knowledge of immortality.
> Om, peace, peace, peace.

Chapter 26

Asteya: There's Plenty to Go Around

I prefer to earn it. It makes me appreciate it more.

....

SONYA TECLAI, AUTHOR OF *NOTES TO SELF*

The yamas are sometimes defined as restraints, ways to pull back on human tendencies that can go awry. *Asteya*, non-stealing, might seem like a write-off because not many of us are shoplifters or safe crackers. Still, we can all get a bit shady when we think there's not enough. Beyond the recipe posted without attribution or the pen we picked up somewhere, asteya suggests that we can steal a host of intangibles: another person's peace, their self-esteem, their turn at being in the spotlight.

We are also invited in asteya to refrain from taking anything not freely offered to us—filching a fry from a spouse's plate, for example. In addition, given the precarious state of the environment at this juncture, it is essential to avoid stealing from Mother Earth and future generations by overusing resources. As Dr. Albert Schweitzer wrote, "That man is truly ethical who shatters no ice crystal as it sparkles in the sun, tears no leaf from a tree."

Unless someone has a mental disorder that predisposes them to steal for the sake of stealing, people most often take from others when they don't have something they need (or want) and don't see any other way to get it. The stealing done by those of us drawn to yoga and spiritual books is more subtle. Our challenge is proactive asteya, establishing ourselves in the conviction that there is indeed plenty to go around: plenty of stuff, attention, love, joy, and time.

Asteya and stuff. One of the blessings of maturity is that very often cravings for possessions diminish. It's a values shift: we start to esteem peace, comfort, service, philanthropy, and free time, as well those classic senior values of health and family, more than acquiring additional belongings and tending to their upkeep. We can further practice asteya around what we believe we are entitled to, e.g., "Mom should have left that ring to me, not my brother who won't appreciate it." Yoga teaches that what is ours will find us and what is not ours won't. But here is the amazing thing: accepting this opens the way for bounty. Patanjali himself writes in verse 2.37 of the Yoga Sutras: "When established in asteya, all jewels appear." In other words, when we stop stealing from others, even in fantasy, prosperity beats a path to our door.

Asteya and attention. We go against asteya when we steal somebody else's thunder. For example, a coworker tells a personal story, and we chime in with "Wait till you hear what happened to me." Or it's a friend's birthday, and we do most of the talking. Or a book club buddy is excited to share that their granddaughter was accepted by a great college, and we chime in that our grandson is going there, too—*with a full scholarship.* As we build our self-worth through spiritual living, we can stop chasing the limelight, do our best work, and let the citrus illumination find us when it's supposed to.

Asteya and love. This one is tough because unlike a fancy car or a dream vacation, we need love at a soul level and every other level. Some older people seem steeped in it: they've been married for decades. Their kids have kids, and everybody's spouse is more like another child than an in-law. They are close to their neighbors, closer to their friends, and everybody thinks the world of them. If we're not in that situation, it is easy to feel cheated and want what they have. Asteya suggests that, instead, we rejoice in what they have and appreciate what we have.

Gratitude is high-powered fertilizer. Sprinkle enough of that stuff on your one good friend, your cousin in Manitoba, and your building's maintenance guy who'll fix anything for you, and you're apt to get two powerful results. First, you will come to see how genuinely precious those three people are, and you can watch as slowly but surely, more loving, caring human beings enter your life.

I experienced this after moving to New York City from the Midwest. During my first year as a New Yorker, I'd made only one really close friend, the late Jay Mulvaney, author of *Jackie and Diana: Maidens, Mothers, Myths*. On the first day of my second year here, I resolved to endlessly appreciate Jay and also to trust that he wasn't the only soul sibling for me in the five boroughs. Within hours, an email showed up telling me about "peace study groups" in private homes around the country. I clicked on New York, expecting that there might be a group in Buffalo or Albany, but there was one in Manhattan, held in an apartment across the street from mine. I could look out my window and into the window of the group's host, Linda Ruocco, a fan of St. Francis and teacher of *A Course in Miracles*. She has now been my friend for over two decades.

Asteya and joy. While it is necessary and important to share fears and sorrows with someone we trust, there is a limit. If we've told the tale to a counselor, a spouse, and our best-ever friend, that's enough. Subsequent rehashes won't change anything, but they will keep us mired in negativity and perhaps steal the joy of the people in whom we're confiding. We might instead spark joy by answering "How are you?" with "Fabulous, how about yourself?" It's not a lie because deep inside, the closer to Truth we get, the more contentment and joy we feel. In later life, if we look only at outer conditions, we could report on all manner of discomforts, slights, and losses. Or we can stick with fabulous and enliven everybody.

Asteya and time. We risk stealing time from others when we make a phone call and start talking without asking first if the callee is free. We steal time when we show up late to a doctor's appointment, a lunch date, or a yoga class. We also do it when we fail to look for the cues that tell us that the other person is done with the conversation or the meeting, even if we would like to extend it.

Time gets tricky with advancing age anyway. When we were both turning 50, a friend told me that this milestone put her in touch with her mortality. I didn't relate one bit. I had a teenage daughter and three stepchildren who were even younger. I was making plans to move to New York City and set the world on fire (in a good way). I saw half my life ahead and it was the better half. I felt similarly at sixty, and that decade turned out to be my best one yet. I wrote a successful book and started a meaningful business. I was traveling, speaking, and podcasting. Because I believe so thoroughly in my work, I felt deeply fulfilled. My inner twenty-something was exhilarated by the life we'd crafted together.

Then came seventy. Just prior to that watershed birthday, my husband had a serious accident. He was released from the hospital as the city was being locked down for the coronavirus pandemic. I lost a good friend and writing mentor to Covid. A year later, I suffered a vaccine reaction. I share this with no political agenda; it is simply what happened to me. I developed chronic fatigue syndrome, and getting past that took intensive ayurvedic treatment. I was no more than out of the woods when William was ailing again, bedridden at home for a month, then hospitalized for surgery and in subacute rehab for another two weeks. As a result, he no longer gets out much, and we've both had to adjust to that. My business moved online and although I show up daily for the brave new world of AI, apps, and algorithms, it's an alien place where I don't expect ever to feel entirely at home.

As I leave my early seventies for the middle ones, time is speeding by. Everybody's grandmother used to say that, and now I know why. At this point, stealing time, literally if it were possible, could be tempting. But we can't steal it. We can only stretch it by getting up early, watching fewer newscasts and more comedies, and responding to life with a rousing "Yes!" even on the days we don't believe we have another yes in us.

PRACTICES FOR THE PATH

As time passes, it can seem that life itself takes more from us than any mugger or pickpocket. When I feel robbed, even a little, I try to remember the part in *Les Misérables* when Jean Valjean, an escapee after nineteen years in prison for nabbing a loaf of bread, steals silver cutlery from the bishop who had given him a night's shelter. When the police apprehend Valjean with the purloined flatware and return with him to the bishop's home, the monsignor says: "I am glad to see you, but how is this? I gave you the candlesticks, too." That is one classy man of the cloth. Anyway, should you ever feel that something is taken from you, you might want to bring those candlesticks to mind.

Chapter 27

Brahmacharya: Sexuality, Spirituality, Seniority

Sex is like everything else in yoga, darling—
slowly, slowly, slowly.

....

STELLA CHERFAS, YOGA TEACHER, AT AGE NINETY-EIGHT

All religions and spiritual teachings weigh in on sex and sexuality with the intention of protecting people from misuse of this powerful energy. All too often, however, harsh judgments are rendered and one-size-fits-all edicts proffered on something that is intensely personal. Yoga includes teachings about sex (and about lack of it: one definition of brahmacharya is celibacy). Advanced yogis, one-pointed in their quest for Self-realization, put all their focus and stamina toward this ultimate goal. They may renounce the world, family, and possessions, choosing the path of the renunciate, a life of chastity.

But it gets complicated, as always seems to be the case with human sexuality. There have been numerous reports of sexual misconduct among ostensibly celibate gurus, suggesting that repression of natural urges is never a good idea. Yoga teaches that with concentrated spiritual work over time, all desire disappears except the desire to unite with God. Of course, many women find that their libido dries up after menopause and it has nothing to do with God. Like I said, it's complicated.

Coming from the same culture as the Kama Sutra, yoga is not prudish. Beyond its moral teaching that we are not to harm others in a sexual way, yoga is concerned with energy, how much we have and what we do with it. Yoga has long viewed orgasm—male orgasm, the only one the ancient teachers were paying attention to—as a way to lose vital energy that could be conserved for spiritual growth, awakening kundalini, opening the chakras, and being freed from the cycle of birth and death. Wow, that could scare a person sexless!

Contemporary science comes at this from a different perspective. In her book, *Rewind Your Body Clock*, Jayney Goddard, president of the Complementary Medical Association (UK), reports that sex, like all exercise, is an antidepressant. Orgasms boost the body's manufacture of the neurotransmitters that lead to better self-image and self-esteem, and by stimulating reward centers in the brain, they reinforce and strengthen memory. Being without a partner does not preclude these benefits. "Research has shown," Goddard writes, "that no matter how an orgasm comes about, it is still a profoundly youth-promoting phenomenon."

Whether you're more concerned about awakening kundalini or fabricating neurotransmitters, the issue of sex for mature people breaks down to (a) love (or genuine caring) and (b) practicality. When sexual expression is a way to show love or sincere care to a partner and receive that for us, it's a glorious thing. The practicality comes when we're looking at issues like erectile dysfunction (an early sign of clogged arteries: cut out the saturated fat) and sexual desire discrepancy. That's a real thing with initials: SDD. It means that one partner is as feisty as ever and the other couldn't get aroused by a closeout sale at the vibrator store. Hopefully, when functionality and compatibility are issues, the people involved can hold fast to the love and caring: loving themselves and honoring their own needs, caring for each other and seeking to understand their partner's needs.

While some very elderly people enjoy sex with surprising frequency, the research indicates that loss of sexual desire takes place in the vast majority of people as they age. For women, this can start in the late forties; for men, it often doesn't happen until their sixties or seventies. In a relationship, this is a substantial gap. Communication, cuddling, and counseling can be invaluable in bridging it. Asana practice can also be advantageous since it brings awareness to the body and a greater understanding of what it can do and what it requires.

Of course, every situation is different. You might not be in a relationship but still desire sexual intimacy. Or perhaps you don't desire sexual intimacy but are looking for companionship. Either circumstance could bring you to the world of senior dating: better than middle school, I'm told, but not by much. Humor can be a great gift here. Another is simply to be interested in other people. You don't have to fall in love, or even in lust, to find someone utterly fascinating.

Moreover, for brahmacharya to be fully relevant outside a monastery, we must look to its second definition, moderation, not only in sexual activity but in every aspect of life. (Note that this means moderation in all beneficial things. There is the temptation to use "a little won't hurt" to justify indulging in something harmful or destructive. Not a good idea. We are worth so much more than that.) Assess, then, how much time you invest in eating, sleeping, working, serving others, searching for Truth, watching TV, surfing the web. If something is out of proportion, you can practice brahmacharya by getting the imbalanced activity back in its proper place.

This aspect of brahmacharya tasks us with accepting physical reality and its limitations, as we strive toward ultimate reality with its enticing limitlessness. Here and now, we're dealing with the twenty-four-hour day and what we can realistically accomplish in that period. It is an observation of brahmacharya for me, at the age I am and with the responsibilities I have, to accept that I can count on twelve high-energy hours, four others during which I'm functional but not zippy, and eight more that have to go for sleep. If I crowd my calendar, it depletes my reserves and impedes the productivity I'd hoped to amplify.

Modifying or eliminating certain yoga postures when the classic form is no longer appropriate is another way to observe brahmacharya. Even with a posture you can perform fully and flawlessly, this yama suggests not taking it to the end point of your endurance or flexibility. It's in that bit of space between what you are doing and what you could do that you're most eloquently practicing yoga. You do something similar every time you say no to a request that would overfill your day or a purchase that would overfill your closet. Brahmacharya contends that "enough" is abundance. When you find it, you'll be richer than a CEO and as content as a calico cat, lounging before a sunny window.

PRACTICES FOR THE PATH

Sex is one thing. Romance is another. When they coincide, the sparks can rival a meteor shower, but we can fill our lives with romance that may have nothing to do with sex. Do a little writing exercise entitled "What I Find Romantic." You can write sentences or just make a list, for example:

- Walking in the rain
- Walking in the snow
- Bookshops
- Roses
- Ribbons
- Old architecture
- Paris
- Afternoon tea
- Indie cinemas
- Vintage boutiques
- Candles

When you know what you find romantic, set about to live a more romantic life.

Chapter 28

Aparigraha: Enough Already

The art of letting go is one well worth learning.
You end up with more as a result.

....

TIRLOK MALIK, FOUNDER OF HAPPY LIFE YOGA

The final yama, *aparigraha*, means non-greed or non-possessiveness. It guards against both the fiscally focused "greed is good" mentality and the bondage that can come from too much collecting, attachment, or identification with possessions, combined with the refusal to accept that all things come to pass, not to stay. Make a note of the epigraph, though: it says, "You end up with more as a result." Just as non-stealing (chapter 26) opens the portals of plenty, refraining from longing additionally throws wide the way for all you need to come to you.

The plight of extreme hoarders depicts what can happen when *having* becomes an illness. We might see a person with garbage in their kitchen and stacks of the *New York Times* going back to the last century. If we look at these folks through a yogic lens, however, we see that the duplicate items and the purchases with tags still attached are not there to fill a house, but to fill a hole inside the person. We all have empty inner spaces. The challenge of yoga (and of life, for that matter) is to fill them with love and productivity and spirituality. For some people, it's less daunting to make another run to the thrift store.

Aparigraha invites each of us, regardless of the volume of our material goods, to detach and disentangle from the encumbrance of excess, whether it is an excess of stuff we want, stuff we own, or an emotional investment in either. This exquisitely applies to growing older when downsizing often comes unbidden and can be disheartening.

Ayurveda tells us that people with strong kapha or out-of-balance kapha are especially prone to overdo in the procurement department—materially and emotionally. This is not a judgment call because excess is relative. In room design, for instance, a warm, cozy look and feel calls for more pillows and footstools and assorted curiosities than sleek modernism does. There's nothing wrong with cozy unless it gets out of hand and you're tripping over all the footstools.

Just be aware if you're kapha-dominant, or if you find yourself acquiring more than you need during the midwinter-to-spring kapha season, that you can keep this generally genial dosha in balance with warmth, regular exercise, and meals that are on the lighter side. You might even consider a partial fast one day each week when you consume only juices (green and other vegetable juices, with the optional addition of lemon or a little other fruit juice), vegetable broth, and herbal tea. This is a frequent suggestion in yoga, but if it's too extreme, remember ayurveda's gentle cleanse: spiced, stewed apples for breakfast and soothing kitchari for the other two meals. You've got to love a detox that allows for chewing and silverware.

You can also bring aparigraha into your life by regular decluttering. Modern science has shown that people who live amidst clutter have higher levels of cortisol, a marker of inflammation, than those with more order around them. And clutter clearing has been shown to bring about more perceived happiness. "When something comes in, something goes out" and "If you haven't used it in a year, you don't need it" got to be platitudes because of their homespun good sense.

Can books you won't read again be gifted to friends or a library? Can worn-out clothing be exchanged, recycled, or at the very least turned into dustcloths? The clothing piece is especially important if you've fallen prey to the fast-fashion trap, outfitting yourself in cheap but stylish garments, usually manufactured in sweatshops and not meant to last. If you pare down to a few great pieces, well made and flattering, and fill in with basics, such as t-shirts and leggings, you'll find yourself developing that look of effortless style that seems to come naturally to Parisians.

Beyond the number of items we own, however, aparigraha is concerned with how attached we are to each one. I don't have much stuff. I moved a lot earlier in life, which kept things from accumulating, and the urban condo where we live now simply cannot accommodate many extras. Even so, I sometimes fall in love with a thing: the white shirt that gets a stain, the pottery bowl that breaks. "Why can I never keep the things I'm most attached to?" I've asked more than once. Eventually, that question answered itself: "Because you're so attached." Aha! It's nonattachment then, not the weight or the worth of our possessions, that is at the core of aparigraha. It's not nearly as much about what we have as what we value.

And lest this looks like a free ride for minimalists, we can become attached to intangibles too: the way we look, what people think of us, a position we've taken on some issue, the interface of a website that worked fine last week but now they've gone and changed it. Because everything in the material universe is in constant flux, we can be at peace only when we allow the world around us to pass by, adapting and amending as it goes. We get to delight in every nanosecond of *now*, as long as we don't try to hold on to it. Mystical poet William Blake stated this perfectly: "He who binds himself to a joy/ Doth its winged life destroy./ He who kisses the joy as it flies/ Lives in eternity's sunrise."

PRACTICES FOR THE PATH

To stay on top of excess, make decluttering part of your yogic lifestyle overall. You can even make a mini retreat of it. Decide which space or spaces you'll tackle and get up early (which we're already doing, right?) to get to it. As part of your morning meditation, set an intention—called a *sankalpa* in yoga—to part with whatever you don't need and rediscover the beauty and usefulness of everything you're keeping. Every few hours, move from outer concerns to inner reflection with twenty minutes of asana and pranayama, or by getting outside to walk and breathe or maybe futz a bit in your garden. At the end of the day, give yourself an A for aparigraha.

Part Eight

Personal Disciplines

Chapter 29

Saucha: Keep It Clean

Cleanliness becomes more important when godliness is unlikely.

....

P.J. O'ROURKE

The yamas we just explored are yoga's don'ts: don't lie, don't steal, and so forth. The *niyamas*, personal disciplines or calls to action, are the to-do list, zeroing in on our private habits. Apart from the niyama regarding cleanliness—we'll explore that one in this chapter—we could ignore these and no one would be the wiser. For our growth and our soul, however, that would be counterproductive, because we build inner strength with these "virtuous observances" the way a bodybuilder bulks up at the gym.

Saucha covers cleanliness, and we will start close to home, with cleanliness of the body. While at least one daily bath or shower is recommended, neither yoga nor ayurveda is a great fan of soap. Certainly, use it for your feet, underarms, and groin area, or if you've been in some serious dirt, but otherwise plain water should be sufficient.

Both yoga and ayurveda offer practices for physical cleansing that go beyond the bath. We covered some of these, such as splash (the face), swish (the mouth), and scrape (the tongue) in chapter 13, "First Thing in the Morning." Others include nasal cleansing with a neti pot, and *garshana*, sluffing off dead skin with a rough glove or dry body brush (see sidebars for both). Yoga also suggests wearing clean clothes daily and even reserving the clothing to be worn during asana and meditation for these uses only. Some practitioners make a discipline of wearing white, either for yoga or all the time, because the act of wearing clothing that "shows the dirt" calls for an added degree of mindfulness.

NASAL CLEARING

When I was first learning about yoga, putting water in one's nose seemed decidedly odd, but now ENTs recommend nasal clearing with a neti pot to remedy dry sinus passages, congestion, and allergy symptoms. To prepare, place comfortably warm, purified water and a level quarter teaspoon of the very fine salt designed for this use in your pot, and stir until dissolved. It is essential that you use distilled or previously boiled water to avoid the low but real risk of serious infection from tap water. It's also important to keep the pot clean. While you can buy plastic neti pots in most drugstores, I recommend a ceramic version that can be washed in the dishwasher or put in a microwave to disinfect before using. To perform nasal irrigation:

- Lean over a basin and bend so that the side of your head is parallel to the floor (this will prevent the saltwater from going into your mouth).
- Inhale *before* you place the spout at the opening of your upper nostril so it can flow into your nasal passage as you exhale, allowing the saltwater to flow out the other side.
- Stand up and gently blow your nose.
- Repeat the process with the other nostril.

Most instructions tell you to use one pot of warm saltwater per nostril; I usually get by with one pot for both. Using a neti pot can take a bit of acclimation but it should be fairly comfortable. To make it even more so, add half a dropperful of Neti Wash Plus, from the Himalayan Institute, also a source for the special salt intended for use in a neti pot. In my experience, the herbal extracts in Neti Wash Plus make the water feel gentler somehow and the process more appealing.

DRY SKIN BRUSHING

In traditional ayurveda, garshana, sloughing off dry surface skin on the body, is done with a raw silk glove, but a plant-fiber dry skin brush that you can find at a natural food store or good pharmacy works just as well. You can do dry skin brushing on its own or, preferably, before abhyanga when freshly brushed skin will drink up the oil, and vata dosha, stimulated by this active process, will balance out with the subsequent oil massage. Start with your feet, and brush toward the heart (although I must admit to doing some back and forth and up and down). Be gentle around your breast area, skip your face entirely, and if you have any kind of skin eruption, such as eczema, avoid those areas. Since the skin's natural sloughing-off process slows with age, dead cells can cause the skin on legs, arms, and elsewhere to become rough and flaky. Dry skin brushing takes care of this. It also helps prevent lymph stagnation and is a particular boon for kapha conditions such as low energy, congestion, and cellulite.

Moving from the body we live in to our living spaces, we got a head start on an inviting environment when we cut down on possessions with aparigraha. Saucha deals with how much dust is on the possessions we kept. We will focus on home, but this also goes for the car, the office, whatever space is ours to use and ours to keep tidy. I'm grateful that cleaning can be spiritual practice, because otherwise I'd like it even less. Seeing it as tending to God's property helps. So does cleaning with music. Gospel, country (I love the stories), Broadway (I love the stories!), and the popular music of my youth all energize my cleaning efforts. (A note on that youth music: researcher Rudolph Tanzi, PhD, and his colleagues at Harvard discovered that when dementia patients listen to the music that was popular in their teens and early twenties, memories are stirred and brain activity triggered.)

But back to cleaning. Like so much else in yoga and life, doing a little every day is essential. Then what you do weekly and seasonally is less arduous. It is also yogic to use cruelty-free and non-toxic products.

Recognizable brands such as Method, Attitude, Mrs. Meyer's Clean Day, and Bon Ami are easy to find in stores and online, and you can do a lot with baking soda, club soda, and white vinegar. Even when using gentle products, I like to open the windows when I clean and let nature do her part. When a counterproductive thought creeps in ("I shouldn't have to be doing this"), I try to remember pratipaksha bhavana and replace that with "I'm grateful to be able to do this."

Finally, there is what my friend Camille DeAngelis calls in her eponymous book about creativity, *A Bright, Clean Mind*. To maintain that kind of mental state asks for a periodic cleanup of both the thoughts we think (see chapter 17) and the messaging we allow in. My husband can watch suspenseful, violent movies just for entertainment. He says they don't affect him at all, and maybe they don't. They affect me as if I myself were living the onscreen apocalypse. I would dump twenty pounds of potting soil onto my living room rug before I would put images like those into my psyche.

Ditto with overconsumption of the news. I have mentioned this before but it bears repeating. I remember, and perhaps you do, too, when civilization persisted with only half an hour of televised news every evening. Just because we can now immerse ourselves in it round the clock, and then find out via social media what everyone else thinks about what happened, does not mean we have to. We know what's going on. World events and pop culture permeate our psychic atmosphere. Saucha says: clean it up. Take in less negativity. Respond in some productive way to the negativity you know about and surrender the rest to All That Is. Keep a journal: it's like having a private landfill for confusion and worry. And meditate daily: The vibrations it generates "clean" the atmosphere where you do it. I believe they ripple out, and like one of those self-steering vacuums, suck up little scraps of sadness as they go.

PRACTICES FOR THE PATH

Thankfully, one of yoga's gifts is that it's not about stringent rules but rather about adapting concepts to work in our lives. With saucha, you can set goals that inspire you, if not the organizing guru du jour. Maybe it is making the bed every day, or getting the dishes done after dinner and unloading the dishwasher each morning so the day's pots and pans and plates won't stack up in the sink. Perhaps it is putting the laundry away as soon as it comes off the line or out of the dryer, or unpacking within twenty-four hours of every trip. This isn't about becoming a clean freak but rather having respect for yourself and the surroundings that influence your mood.

Chapter 30

Santosha: All Is Well

At some point, you gotta let go, and sit still, and allow contentment to come to you.

....

ELIZABETH GILBERT

Contentment, *santosha* in Sanskrit, is the new euphoria. It has a much longer shelf life. A reminder to be content with present-moment reality, this niyama does not prevent us from making changes in our lives or in society. It rather enables us to be at peace with the progress we've made to date and live harmoniously with the unsolved problems that are part and parcel of life on earth.

As mature yogis, we have some unique opportunities to observe santosha. For starters, we can be content with what we're able to accomplish on the mat—or in chair yoga class if getting up from the floor is no longer a reasonable request. There are postures I never mastered, notably those calling for a lot of upper body strength, and others that I could once do but not any longer. The wheel, yoga's full backbend, is one of those: my wrists simply don't bend that far backwards anymore. I could resent that and get depressed about it, or force it and cause an injury, or go with santosha, accept the way things are, and focus on other options: bridge pose, locust, boat, bow.

Another very present opportunity older people have to embrace santosha is with technology. Not being able to talk to a customer service rep, or get into an account without unearthing an inexplicably altered password, can cause genuine angst for people who lived rich lives for decades without these aggravations. Santosha says that we don't have to be great fans of the way things are, only that we be at peace with the way things are. It's like Iris said all those years ago, "the darling physical plane." It is just that now, navigating the darling physical plane requires passwords. Before long, I'm sure, it will be something else.

Whatever the particulars, santosha calls for looking within and getting our bearings there. If we can't be content without sunshine, a bull market, and attentive adult children, our priceless serenity goes out of our control. The Bhagavad Gita expounds on this exquisitely when Lord Krishna, believed to be, like Jesus, an incarnation of the Infinite, shores up the resolve of his cousin, Arjuna, a soldier whose duty is to fight in a battle he dreads. At one point, Krishna tells Arjuna, "Those who are alike in happiness and distress. . .who accept both blame and praise with equanimity. . .who remain the same in honor and dishonor. . .they are said to have risen above the three gunas." In other words, the exigencies of the material world no longer get to them. It's a lofty goal, but santosha, practicing contentment in any circumstance, brings us closer.

Personally, I have had a hard time with this one. It's tempting to get up and let my phone tell me the state of the weather, the state of the world, the length of my to-do list, and the number of my commitments. My brain calculates these and gives me a rating for the day before it even starts. On a scale of one to ten—well, it's never a ten. When instead I keep those first couple of hours sacrosanct, focused on inner work and self-care, I am able to build a base of contentment not likely to be shaken by what's on my calendar or in the headlines.

Finding joy in sweet simplicities also boosts santosha. Remember the ayurvedic suggestion in chapter 13 to give each of your senses some tiny delight first thing in the morning? For me, the most delightful is often little Rupert, our rescue dog. He has PTSD, coming as he did from animal hoarding, and seeing him each day get more and more in touch with his inner dog makes everything else seem possible too. Then there is William's good morning. The familiarity of the yoga mat. The luxurious indulgence of abhyanga, warm oil massage. The sacred gift of meditation. The aromatic excellence of the ginger, cardamom, nutmeg, cinnamon, and clove on my oatmeal at breakfast.

Throughout the day I remind myself: go within first. Yes, I have to look outside to determine the time, the train schedule, somebody else's mood. And I'm fully willing to revel in jubilation from a surprise, a serendipity, somebody's saying something really nice, something I'd hoped would happen happening. Even so, santosha tells me to cherish contentment whether rapture shows up or not, and to maintain that contentment after a run-in with elation that then fades away, as it always does.

Did I mention that I have not yet mastered this? Good, because if you talk to my friends or, heaven forbid, my husband, they will set you straight. That's why santosha, like everything else about yoga, is a *practice.* Helping me to practice santosha these days is the favorite combo-affirmation of the late Louise Hay. Known as an author, publisher, and affirmation expert, Hay was also a great role model for aging well. A sixty-four-year-old cancer survivor when her classic, *You Can Heal Your Life,* was published, Hay came to prominence in what we call the retirement years. She died in her sleep at age ninety. Here's the affirmation: "All is well. Everything is working out for my highest good. Out of this situation only good will come. I am safe."

I typed it up and printed it—I'm of the paper generation—and hung copies around the apartment so I would read these statements a lot. As various problems cropped up and I'd say that third sentence, "Out of this situation only good will come," I'd add in my mind or under my breath, "Yeah, right." But you know what? She was right. This world isn't perfect. My life isn't perfect. And whoever was first to say "Old age isn't for sissies" was spot-on. Still, things work out a high percentage of the time, and you and I have both been observing life long enough to know that our attitude can affect that percentage.

PRACTICES FOR THE PATH

Call on santosha when the piddly stuff threatens to rob your peace. You may have observed, as I have, that we can show great poise in a crisis, while our response to misplacing the keys or spilling a coffee may be less than exemplary. Set the intention for yourself that every minor irritation will remind you to remember santosha, cling to contentment, and maybe even laugh about that lapse with the latté.

Chapter 31

Tapas: Boot Camp for Yogis

*The whole science of character building may be regarded as
a practice of tapas.*

....

B.K.S. IYENGAR

This chapter could be about Spanish appetizers. It isn't. In yoga, *tapas* means discipline, but before I lose you, this isn't punishment. It is more like training for an athletic event or studying for an advanced degree: rugged, difficult, and sometimes you want to give up. If you don't give up, that's tapas.

Sometimes referred to as *inner fire*, tapas applies to both the "austerities" we might impose upon ourselves, such as early nights, early mornings, and daily yoga practice, and to the boldness and grit we need to face what life hands out. When I think of tapas, I always hear one of my yoga teachers, Dhyana Masla, saying, "Life is not happening *to* you. It's happening *for* you." When we really get that, we no longer need to avoid or outwit the hard stuff, because it's no longer all that intimidating.

Tapas has a long history. Centuries before the codification of raja yoga by Patanjali, spiritual aspirants put themselves through all kinds of hardships to reach enlightenment. Sometimes they overdid it, as Gautama, who became the Buddha, realized when he saw that years of fasting and deprivation had weakened his body more than they had strengthened his being. He went on to develop the Middle Path of good-sense spirituality now called Buddhism.

A reasonable practice of yoga is a middle path too. To include tapas in it, we incorporate a task or a test that inspires us. It needs to be sufficiently doable that we'll do it, but demanding enough that we will at times be tempted to amend or avoid it. It is in that place of wanting to abandon ship but sticking with it that the fire of transformation ignites, burning away some unwanted foible or an old pattern called in yoga a *samskara*. Everything we do and everything that happens to us leaves an impression. The changing colors of leaves in autumn may spark the connection "back to school." If we loved school and did well there, that's a positive samskara; if we were bullied or struggled with dyslexia, the resulting samskara is likely to cause angst. Tapas can help do away with some of the negative impressions and fill the void with a higher degree of character and resolve.

Advancing age presents opportunities to rev up that inner fire as we experience changes and losses we'd opt out of if we could. Facing them is tapas in action. If you're dealing with a chronic illness, you're a caregiver, or living in an expensive world on a limited income, I would not expect you to give up Sunday brunch simply to make things more onerous. (You might, however, get in a little tapas by committing to walk one way.) If, on the other hand, you are feeling that life is pretty cushy and you could use a shakeup, stretch yourself. Train for a race. Let go of wine with dinner—if not forever, for some predetermined period. This is personal. If I were going to plot out some tapas propositions for the year ahead, my list would look like this:

- *Do what scares you first.* (As someone who must watch out for excess vata, fear and procrastination can be issues for me.)
- *No screens before 9 a.m. or after 9 p.m.* (I'm usually pretty good about this, but making it a tapas challenge would get rid of "usually" and "pretty.")
- *Do the nighttime dog walk promptly at 8.* (It's cold. It's dark. If I wait long enough, maybe someone will knock on the door to volunteer. But of course they won't.)
- *Arrive ten minutes early.* (I'm always either right on time or a couple of minutes late, and didn't we say in the chapter on

asteya that lateness robs time from other people? It also adds to stress and aggravates vata. That ten-minute tapas could be a game changer.)

So, maybe I *have* made my tapas plans going forward. Hopefully my list inspires yours. You can also take a prompt from the Bhagavad Gita, noting that tapas comes in three categories: body, speech, and mind.

- *Tapas of the body* does not refer only to athletic challenges or avoiding some item of food or drink, but also to those things we do in a physical way to relate to others, help others, or engage actively in worship or devotion. You might resolve to take part in a weekly group meditation, do volunteer work, or take over one of your spouse's chores for the month of their birthday.
- *Tapas of speech* can be a commitment to speak positively, refrain from demeaning self-talk, or take a moratorium on gossip. If you think you don't gossip, how about trying a week when you don't mention third parties at all, even in a neutral or complementary way? Or you might swear off swearing. The pinnacle of tapas in terms of speech, however, is a silence fast for a day or a weekend. You can even sign up for a silent retreat of a week or longer. It is an experience everyone should have at least once. While most people who do this report experiencing a depth of peace and a buildup of energy reserves they would never have expected, the Gita is clear that we're not to engage in tapas with the thought of reaping a reward.
- *Tapas of the mind* deals with thinking the highest, purest thoughts you can, and gently noticing when you fall shy of this. You might choose to double up on meditation, or select an affirmation, quotation, or piece of scripture and contemplate its meaning for a prescribed period each day. You could also pray for others or hold them in your highest thoughts. A powerful suggestion in the book, *Alcoholics Anonymous*, is to pray daily for one month that some person you resent manifest in their life

precisely what you want in yours. The lightening of soul that comes from doing this is beyond description.

Tapas offers a lot to choose from, even if you never go so far as laying off chocolate.

PRACTICES FOR THE PATH

Come up with your own tapas list. A few of your entries can be changes you want to make permanent, and others can be exercises set to last for some limited period. Spans people tend to choose are one, three, seven, ten, twenty-one, thirty, and forty days——Lent can be a stunning time for tapas.

Chapter 32

Svadhyaya: Study of the Self and the Sacred

Re-examine all you have ever been told.
Dismiss what insults your soul.

....

WALT WHITMAN

When Tevye sings "If I Were a Rich Man" in *Fiddler on the Roof*, he says that what he wants most to do is "sit in the synagogue and pray...discuss the holy books...several hours every day." I don't know of a yogi who has expressed *svadhyaya*, study of the self and the sacred, better than he did. This observance is precisely what Tevye craves. It is first turning inward to find who's there, and then, for Tevye and for yogis, comes study of sacred texts. This niyama addresses the studious side of yoga and the importance of making time for it every day, whether or not you happen to be a rich man.

Yoga has no corner on the quest for self-knowledge: the Delphic oracle made a billboard of it. Yoga's version, however, is that we seek to know the various aspects of ourselves until we reach the ultimate reality, that Self beyond the body, mind, ego, and personality. On the way, we can discover fascinating information about our body, mind, ego, and personality, about the meaning of past experiences and the way to best steer our lives going forward. It is paradoxical that, at the root of everything, we are not separate at all, but in our present reality we are unique, and learning about our uniqueness will help us along our journey. "Study thy self, discover the divine," Patanjali states in Yoga Sutra 2.44.

There are untold ways to learn about ourselves. You did it when you took the dosha quiz, and you do it if you keep a journal. Especially when you write with a pen instead of a keyboard, free writing intended for no eyes but your own can be quite revealing. Ditto observing yourself while on your yoga mat. How is your breathing? If it's rapid or shallow, why do you think that is? Where is there tension in your body? Can you release it? Are you fully present to your practice, or is your mind elsewhere? Why?

As you go about your daily doings, how do you see yourself? Where did your opinions about yourself come from? Are some of these childhood assessments you heard once or quite a bit? Are they still accurate? Were they ever? If there is some guilt or regret from the past intruding on today, can you write about it or talk about it and be willing to let it go?

Take a peek at your motivations. Do the resulting actions reflect who you are today, or are you striving by habit for a prize you no longer want? Are you seeking to please someone who no longer needs pleasing? Take some time to contemplate what you do, why you do it, and what you might want to do differently in the future. One technique is, at bedtime, to play your day back like a movie. (The Catholic Ignatian tradition calls this practice the Examen.) Give yourself credit where it's due, and examine with zero judgment any incidents you would rescript if you could—and you can, to a degree at least, by making amends if called for and behaving differently when a similar situation arises, which it will.

"What I've learned from svadhyaya," says yoga instructor and memoirist Sande Nosonowitz, "is to stay curious, to let self-knowledge come by being open to it, and quelling the inner critic enough to discover new things." All this inward turning allows you to notice "the witness," a term you will sometimes see in yogic writings to connote the Self. If you observe yourself doing what you do, who is observing while "you" are busy doing? This is a deep question and an important one. While many answers come from introspection, wise ones who came before us left writings to guide our way.

Therefore, the other aspect of svadhyaya is to study sacred books—and I would add to that any written material that gets you closer to peace than you were before you read it. Nevertheless, scriptures are in a class by themselves, separated by their myriad levels of meaning from writings that are simply astute or inspiring. Their adventurous tales and accessible parables make scriptural teachings available even to children, but layer by layer, beneath and beneath, scripture reveals ever deeper truths. This is why a person can devote a lifetime to studying a single one and never tire of it.

Within the yoga tradition, and the Hindu religion, is the aforementioned Bhagavad Gita, part of a breathtaking epic of power and intrigue, the Mahabharata. The other great Indian saga is the Ramayana, an engrossing allegory interwoven with moral and philosophical teachings. Other texts of scriptural status include the Yoga Sutras of Patanjali, the Hatha Yoga Pradipika, and the Upanishads, early writings dealing with meditation, philosophy, and the nature of being and consciousness. But scriptures have come to us from the world over, and if the Bible, the Quran, the Guru Granth Sahib, the Tao Te Ching, the Dhammapada, or something else speaks to you, your study of that is svadhyaya.

You might ask, "How could that be? Don't they all say different things?" Yes, in some respects, on the surface. They're like us that way. In outward expression, we are diverse individuals who can disagree with one another on just about anything, and yet deep, deep within, we are the One Life. The world's holy books come from sundry times, places, and cultures. They come in different translations and appeal to different people, but the spirit that embodies and infuses them is that One Life too.

When Mahatma Gandhi died, his possessions were, in total, the dhoti he wore, a pair of sandals, his eyeglasses, and one copy each of the Bhagavad Gita and the New Testament. It seems that even before digital devices, all the wisdom of the universe could fit in a pocket.

PRACTICES FOR THE PATH

Sometimes we can best come to know ourselves by exploring the lives and contributions of others. Look at the biography section in the "Brilliant Books" bibliography, and check out these documentaries:

- *Awake: The Life of Yogananda* highlights important developments in the life of the yogi who came to America in the 1920s and made sure we'd never forget.

- *What Is Real? The Story of Jivamukti Yoga* looks at its visionary founders, Sharon Gannon and David Life, their artistic beginnings, and the influence of their three gurus.

- *Fierce Grace* is the moving film that follows American yogi Ram Dass after a massive stroke at age sixty-five. I know of no better presentation of applying spiritual principles to life's trials than this. "The stroke wasn't bad," Ram Dass said. "It was grace."

Chapter 33

Ishvara Pranidhana: Let Go, Let God

God is peace, bliss, beauty, and truth. Focus your energy on that, life will be like that.

....

AMIT RAY, MEDITATION MASTER

If a Twelve-Step Program is part of your journey, you will recognize this niyama calling for surrender to the Divine as a yogic rendition of the third step, which reads, "We made a decision to turn our will and our lives over to the care of God as we understood Him." (Change the pronoun if you like; a lot of people do.) Twelve-steppers are terrific role models for seeing this kind of surrender not as losing or giving up, but as giving over to a Higher Power of one's own understanding the burden of an insurmountable trial. The Twelve Steps showed up in 1935 but the same message came to the Biblical Psalmist thousands of years earlier: "Cast your burden on the Lord and he will sustain you." *Ishvara pranidhana* is Patanjali's saying the same thing in his Yoga Sutras.

I love this niyama, probably because it was, in its step three iteration, largely responsible for liberating me from the binge eating disorder that ravaged my life into my thirties. In some ways, it is a gift to face an obstacle so enormous that you have to do something gloriously drastic. Surrender is harder when things seem to be going just fine, but yoga teaches that "just fine" applies only when your spiritual growth is proceeding unhindered. In other words, even if there is no pressing need for you to surrender all you are, have, and do to some Divinity you're not sure exists, try it anyway. Patanjali promises that this single act can be a guarantee of reaching that state of union that the very word "yoga" implies.

While every aspect of the yogic journey is designed to help us overcome internal hindrances to progress and peace, this one is singularly capable of taking on all our barriers to enlightenment, called *kleshas* in Sanskrit, in one fell swoop. These kleshas are *avidya*: ignorance, delusion; *asmita*: attachment to the ego; *raga*: attachment to everything else—power, pleasure, cash and prizes; *dvesha*: aversion to (and avoidance of) what we find unpleasant; and *abhinivesha*, fear of death (just to throw in an easy one). If you look at that list, you see the human condition spelled out. If these were eradicated from our species, there would be no prejudice or war or environmental destruction. But since we can't do a klesha-ectomy on other people, we would do well to implement Ishvara pranidhana in our personal sphere.

If you are someone who has a concept of a Higher Power that you're fond of, you can do this forthwith. It's a colossal relief, like setting down a heavy piece of furniture once it's moved to where it's supposed to be. *Ishvara* means Lord, the Divine in a personal sense, as opposed to Brahman, the Absolute, impersonal essence of everything. *Pranidhana* means to surrender or dedicate. That is the verb, the action word. The magic is in the surrender. Your concept of the Infinite is your business. And if that happens to be nothing, not a problem: surrender to taking the high road, listening to your inner voice, or simply following these instructions in the spirit of scientific inquiry. If the result proves the principle, you are no longer asking yourself to believe in anything, because now you know.

You can do this alone, perhaps in front of your altar, simply putting the Divine in charge of things the way you'd make another person host of a Zoom meeting. Or a friend can be part of it. My most recent Ishvara pranidhana experience was with a spiritual sister in a breathtaking Anglican church, circa 1868, here in Manhattan. You can't very well forget an intention you set in the presence of all that stained glass. But here's the thing: the initial "This is cool, I'm going with God" experience is a lot like a wedding: "Love, honor, and cherish—you betcha."

Committing to the practice daily is a marriage: loving and cherishing on the days when Prince or Princess Charming isn't charming at all, when instead of stained glass, you are looking at a dirty window. Fear not: you can re-remember every day or a dozen times a day. "Oops! I dedicated my life to a Higher Power. Let's fix what I just did and start over."

And when you do—over and over and over and over if you're like me—it gets easier. You start to feel that something is working in and for your life, something in addition to your own (very necessary) efforts. You find yourself less alone and less afraid. It's easier to be loving, because you feel so incredibly loved, for always and forever, no matter what.

PRACTICES FOR THE PATH

Mention was made of "your altar." If you don't have one, it is worthy interior design for your interior life. Your altar will reflect you, and you can change it at will. Generally speaking, altar attire includes objects and images of spiritual significance to you: pictures or statues of holy people, religious symbols, candles, incense, stones, fresh flowers (replaced before they start to droop), or reminders of special memories. Many people put their altar in a meditation room or corner. Some have an altar in every room. I have one, a shelf in a bookcase I can see from my bed. Among its contents is a pinecone given me by Horus, a very impressive evergreen I met (and named) on a labyrinth walk last summer. At the center of my altar is a picture of Christ meditating with animals when, as legend has it, he traveled to the Himalayas during his lost years. I don't know that this happened, but the image resonates with me, whether it did or whether it didn't.

Part Nine

The Soul of Yoga

Chapter 34

Pratyahara: Give Your Senses a Rest

Yoga has a sly, clever way of short circuiting the mental patterns that cause anxiety.

....

BAXTER BELL, MD

The list of moral precepts (Part Seven) and the personal disciplines (Part Eight), as well as physical postures and breathwork (chapters 6 and 7), are the four active practices of the eight limbs of yoga. In this section, we will look at the second four limbs, the more internal elements. Because our physical being and the subtler aspects of ourselves are intimately connected, what we do with one affects the other. In terms of aging well, all these are believed to produce extended youthfulness and liveliness. The ones more spiritual in nature need never be modified or scaled back to accommodate an aging body, because the soul isn't counting.

Equal in yogic standing to asana or meditation is *pratyahara*, "withdrawal of the senses." It is often overlooked, however, because it can be a difficult concept to grasp. It was like that for me until the morning I decided to walk home from Penn Station. I was listening to Dr. David Frawley's book, *Yoga and Ayurveda*, on Audible, and he'd just come to his exposition of pratyahara as I approached Times Square. Dwarfed by giant action billboards, and in the noisy crossfire of horns, sirens, and an Elmer Gantry wannabe preaching hellfire through a bullhorn, I started to laugh. The universe had captured my attention: "You're not clear on pratyahara? Well, this is what it *isn't*."

Yoga calls the standard five senses "cognitive" and adds to these "active senses," including speaking and moving. In pratyahara, we temporarily accept less sensory input through our eyes, ears, nose, tongue, or skin, or we voluntarily still the voice or the body. Fasting from all food or certain foods is a ubiquitous religious discipline that a yogi would see as pratyahara. While it has a place in tapas, too (chapter 31), observing silence for a day, a weekend, or more, is classic pratyahara. Simply putting yourself in a quiet environment for even a few minutes is a way to observe this.

A compelling pratyahara practice in the contemporary world is to keep an electronic sabbath: choosing a day each week when you enjoy life without TV, computer, or smartphone. It's tough when we depend on our phones for communication, directions, information, scheduling, fitness tracking, and entertainment. We may even count on them to wake us up for Brahma muhurta, hear morning affirmations, participate in an online yoga class, or listen to a lecture from our favorite spiritual teacher or an audiobook expounding on pratyahara.

This is all great stuff, of course, but as Marshall McLuhan astutely determined long before the digital age, "The medium is the message." What we need a break from is not early mornings and asana classes but from the devices that deliver them. For me, an electronic sabbath is a life reset. I can take Rupert to the park or stay home with my husband and remember why we fell in love. I might go to a class or a religious service or shop in an actual store (fitting rooms: what a concept!). I could spend the afternoon talking with one friend about one million things. Now, sometimes I cheat: no computer or TV, but I need the phone. What if the friend I'm meeting needs to reach me? What if I need to check on the hours of that store with the fitting rooms?

We do what we can and what we're willing. All these instructions are to chip away at the concretized beliefs that we are this body and it's getting older, that our worth is tied to what we do, and that if we don't show up on social media for a day, we no longer count. As Richard J. Leider and David A. Shapiro state in their exceptional book, *Who Do You Want to Be When You Grow Old?*—"Whereas the midlife crisis is typically about the loss of opportunities, the late-life crisis is more about the loss of relevance." So, we assert our relevance by posting a nice selfie (camera above eye level, of course; it's more flattering). Most of the time, this is fine. It's fun, and fun is good for every part of us. We are having a life on earth in the twenty-first century, for heaven's sake! Splendid. But sometimes, and you decide when, taking a rest from it is appropriate.

There's a lovely breathing exercise, *bhramari*, the "bumblebee breath," that I intentionally left out of the pranayama chapter to describe it here. In doing bhramari, the mouth is closed, the eyes are held shut with the first two fingers, the ears are shut off with the thumbs, and you hum. I was taught to do this five times, using different pitches for each of the hums. The awareness during bhramari is pure self-containment—and it was the first thing I did when I got home from Times Square.

PRACTICES FOR THE PATH

Back in chapter 3, it was suggested that you select a day each week to put your spiritual life front and center. Can you also make that day an electronic sabbath, fully or partially? If you're someone who spends a lot of time online or watching television, this could be a daunting suggestion. That's all the more reason to try it.

Chapter 35

Dharana, Dhyana, Samadhi: Concentration, Meditation, Connection

Nothing is so aggravating as calmness.

....

MAHATMA GANDHI

The final three limbs of yoga are *dharana*, concentration, *dhyana*, meditation, and *samadhi*, ecstatic union, akin to the mystical experience or beatific vision in Christian tradition, in which the meditation process is sometimes called "contemplative prayer." Of dharana, dhyana, and samadhi, only the first, concentration, is something we can will ourselves to do. Most of what we call meditation is really concentration, bringing the mind back to a focal point: the breath, or an image, word, or phrase on which the mind can center. I'll use the blanket term "meditation" here. Just know that in a true meditative state, our one-pointed awareness is uninterrupted, whether we're sitting cross-legged watching our breath or driving in a blizzard or a downpour when being fully present is nonnegotiable.

In any case, meditation is the Swiss Army Knife of the spiritual life. If you asked me, I'd tell you that I meditate every day—well, nearly—although I sometimes feel more comfortable in saying that I *sit* every day and recall a mantra I chose for myself. "Sitting" is a term often used in Buddhism to connote meditation, this showing up to be still. When I do it, my mind wanders and I invite it back. This happens to everybody because movement is the nature of the mind. Sometimes I think mine wanders more than it used to, now that I'm older and spacey vata leads to flights of fancy. But if I sit and breathe and return my focus when I realize it's somewhere else, that is meditation, allowing the mind to focus on a single point.

There are numerous styles of meditation in the yogic arsenal, but here I will simply share with you what I do: sit silently with a mantra. This is easily customized to individual proclivities—sacred or secular, Sanskrit or not. So, you sit, either in a cross-legged position on the floor, your bed if it's fairly firm, or in a chair; in this case, have both feet on the floor. Leaning against the chair back, the wall, or a sturdy headboard is fine, as long as your spine stays fairly straight.

Invite yourself into the process by watching your inhalations and exhalations several times, giving yourself the suggestion that with each exhalation you're settling more deeply into the process. Then bring in your mantra. *Om shanti*—shanti means peace—is lovely, as is *so hum*, "I am That," a way to identify with Ultimate Reality. It is taught that these Sanskrit words carry power by means of their sound vibration, but if you're more comfortable sticking with English, any simple phrase that appeals to you will work: "Be still and know" or "All is well."

Although there are variations in this technique that you can learn from a teacher or a course or a website, I like to align the mantra and the breath. So, I'd do (inhale) "Om," exhale "shanti." (Or inhale "so," exhale "hum"; inhale "Be still," exhale "and know"; or inhale "All is," exhale "well.") That's all there is to it, except to bring the mind back—Om Shanti, All is well—when it strays. St. Francis of Assisi is credited with saying that thoughts during meditation are like birds flying around your head. It is not a problem that they're there; you just don't want to invite them to build nests in your hair.

How long do you do it? I am tempted to say for as long as you're willing, long enough to touch some peace most days but not so long that it becomes laborious and you quit. To start, ten minutes is probably plenty, but some people get so much out of it that they go on meditation retreats and sit in silence for hours each day. Twenty minutes is the length of time taught to students of the Transcendental Meditation technique, which has been studied longer than any other by scientists to determine the physical and psychological benefits of meditation. TM practitioners use a mantra technique and meditate twice a day, morning and early evening, twenty minutes each time. A late-day meditation is a lovely way to get a second wind after work and clear away any mental detritus accumulated since morning.

Still, many dedicated meditators of other traditions stick with mornings only and reap tremendous benefits. It's fine to open your eyes and check a nearby clock to see what your time is, or set an unobtrusive timer. You can download the Insight Timer app, which will time your meditation and give you a variety of opportunities for spiritual and holistic education and experiences. There's also the Simple Meditation Timer app; all it does is time your meditation, which may be all you need.

It is good not to jump right up from meditation. Ideally, your mind went from the fully wakeful state, characterized by beta brain waves, into an alpha state. Give yourself a minute or a few minutes to recalibrate. Sometimes you'll feel wonderful after meditation: calm, creative, positive, inspired. Other days you'll feel the way you do after brushing your teeth: *Well, that's done.* The benefits accrue either way. If you are doing this for the long haul—moksha, liberation, all knowledge, total bliss, no more births, deaths, or taxes—every session is an investment towards that. You can think of it as the cosmic retirement plan. Or maybe for now you just want to age like a yogi. It works for that too.

In the 1970s, research scientists started taking a serious interest in what effect meditation might have on people physically and emotionally. The preeminent early researcher was Harvard's Herbert Benson, MD, the cardiologist who wrote the groundbreaking book *The Relaxation Response* and was professor emeritus at the Benson-Henry Institute for Mind Body Medicine at Massachusetts General Hospital.

Since then, researchers have looked at meditators six ways to Sunday. Whether practitioners of TM or Insight Meditation, a Buddhist technique that bypasses the mantra and simply observes the breath, subjects invariably show measurable boons. These include reductions in stress, anxiety, and inflammation, improved blood pressure regulation, boosted immunity, fewer sick days, better sleep, and help with pain management and addiction recovery. Exciting research at UCLA showed that regular meditation inhibited the shrinkage of the brain that comes with age. They determined that long-term meditators at fifty had brains seven and a half years "younger" than expected, and the rejuvenation continued at a rate of one month and twenty-two days per year after that. This is, quite literally, aging in reverse.

If you do nothing else to age like a yogi, engage in regular meditation. It may mean silencing your devices, putting a "Do Not Disturb" sign on your door, or getting up for Brahma muhurta to have undisturbed quiet time. Eventually, though, you will be able to meditate even when circumstances are less than idyllic—on public transportation, for example, or in a hospital room with monitors beeping.

And then there is the promise of samadhi, that experience of connection, absorption, of knowing you are part of all that is. Sri Swami Sivananda writes, "Samadhi is an indescribable state. It is beyond the reach of mind and speech. The meditator loses his little individuality and becomes identical with the Supreme Self. He becomes an embodiment of bliss, peace and knowledge."

While I can speak from experience about headstands and alternate nostril breathing, how to do self-massage with warm sesame oil, and the many merits of turmeric, the closest I've come to samadhi is the occasional ecstatic glimpse. Like the "previews of coming attractions" alluded to when we discussed chakras, I'm sure you've experienced this too: a momentary sense of kinship with all life, a powerful awareness of being supported, shored up, and loved with an everlasting love. This impresses the heart like a stamp on a passport, and then the mind returns to the mundane: "I think we're out of peanut butter." Even so, the glimpses tell us that more of these sweet sightings are around the corner.

Sri Patanjali emphasizes tending to this inner quieting "for a long time, without interruption, and with devotion" (Sutra 1.4). If you miss a day, make sure it's not two days. If you stop altogether because of illness or grief or you took a vacation or got into pickleball, return as soon as you notice what's happened. Once again, sit and breathe and invite your mind back when it scampers off. Then do it again. And again. I have never known anyone to regret it.

PRACTICES FOR THE PATH

Don't miss out on this. If it is really intimidating to be with what seems like nothingness, start with something meditative instead of classic meditation. These techniques can be helpful for lapsed meditators as well as cautious newbies. Prayer is a beautiful introduction to meditation and a companion for it: it is often said that prayer is talking to God, and meditation is letting God answer. Praying the rosary, if that is part of your tradition, has meditative focus built in; mala beads, a string of 108 beads designed for repeating the names of God, is another option. Journaling is meditative, too: there is even a meditation technique called *likita japa*, writing a mantra over and over and focusing on the process.

In addition, guided meditations abound on the internet. Purists would object to calling these "meditation" because enough fully awake brain activity goes on while listening to one that you may not reach the alpha state. Even so, they are undeniably inspiring. Immerse yourself in them if they are more appealing right now than straight silence. But don't give up on silence: it will be there for you when you're ready.

Chapter 36

What Kind of Yogi Are You?

What I love about yoga is that it's a science. If we do the practices—meditation, breathwork, asana, chanting, the yamas and niyamas—we get a prescribed result.

....

RADHA METRO-MIDKISS, INTEGRAL YOGA INSTITUTE

We have been exploring *raja yoga*, the royal path, yoga as psychology, presented by Patanjali in his Yoga Sutras. Its goal is to still the mind, and it includes the eight limbs we've touched on: yamas (moral precepts), niyamas (personal disciplines), asana (postures), pranayama (breathwork), pratyahara (withdrawal of the senses), dharana (concentration), dhyana (meditation), and samadhi (divine connection). The process is clearly delineated and serves and satisfies millions. Even so, one size need not fit all. There are types of yoga other than Patanjali's raja, "royal," pathway. One of these may suit you better than all these limbs and lists. You can also add one or more of these yogic treasures to your personal practice. In fact, any practice would be the better for it.

Karma yoga: People are often surprised to learn that the direct translation of karma is "action," not simply the results of our actions, and that there is an action-based path called karma yoga, selfless service. It is ideal for those who will never stop being busy and who would do well to steer that busyness toward the betterment of all. Anyone who looks forward to retirement so they can do volunteer work full-time has the soul of a karma yogi. Some karma yogis that we've heard of, whether or not they would describe themselves as such, include Mahatma Gandhi, Mother Teresa, and Greta Thunberg.

Work becomes karma yoga when it's motivated by the work itself or the spirit of service, rather than payment or praise. While payment may be rendered and praise received, karma yoga has as its essence nonattachment. For example, the attorney who gives the same care and attention to a pro bono case as to one with billable hours is practicing karma yoga. Any full engagement, giving oneself to the task at hand, paid or not, is karma yoga. Work done in this way is a kind of active meditation. While losing oneself in work is not uncommon, karma yogis use labor or service or egoless creative expression to lose themselves in the Infinite.

Bhakti yoga: Bhakti is the yoga of devotion and love, described by twentieth century theologian Dr. Ernest Wilson as ideal for those who do well having a "God with skin on." A bhakta can love Krishna or Jesus, a guru or a goddess, while simultaneously recognizing the sacred in all beings and all creation. This heart-centered path is about a loving relationship with the Divine, and a key tenet is the equality of all people. It intersects here with karma yoga because serving others also serves the Beloved.

Characterized by music, joy, praise, and rapture, with *japa*, repetition of divine names, a key practice, bhakti has been called the most natural form of spirituality. We are, after all, born with the capacity to love others. In addition, we have slumbering within us a deep love for the Divine that yearns to be awakened. Through this love, one can cultivate detachment from the things of this world and develop an enviable equipoise.

A well-known proponent of bhakti was Ram Dass, author of the innovative book, *Be Here Now*. The former Richard Alpert was a Harvard colleague of Timothy Leary's and with him co-pioneered the 1960s psychedelic movement. Alpert later found his spiritual teacher, Neem Karoli Baba, became Ram Dass, and moved from chemically incited mind-altering experiences to truly spiritual ones. Beatle George Harrison was also a bhakta and part of the Hare Krishna movement; if you listen to the lyrics of his "My Sweet Lord," you'll get the gist of bhakti and know if it resonates with you.

Jnana yoga, the path of knowledge via self-analysis, is said to be the shortest, albeit the steepest, way to enlightenment. If we say that karma yogis want most to *do* and bhakti yogis want most to *love*, jnana yogis most what to *know*. A jnani asks, *"What does all this mean? What am I doing here?"* And they ask above all: *"Who am I?"* While the meditation process in other yogas aims to still the mind, jnana meditation is designed to reach the Self beyond the mind. A well-known jnana meditation is *Neti, neti*, "Not this, not that." The meditator asks, "Am I the body?" Neti, neti. "Am I this personality?" Neti, neti. "Am I my possessions?" Neti, neti. "Am I what others think of me?" Neti, neti. "Am I the beliefs I hold?" Neti, neti.

Scientists and engineers are often drawn to this path of self-examination. While enlightenment for a bhakta is to come into full, loving connection with the Divine, enlightenment for a jnani is to come to realize that they and the Divine have been one all along. A word often associated with jnana (and the closely related spiritual system of Vedanta) is *advaita*, nondualism. The implication is that everyone and everything is Brahman, and to know this about ourselves, deeply and genuinely with no whiff of doubt, brings total liberation.

Swami Vivekananda, the first spiritual teacher from India to journey to the West, is generally regarded as a jnani, although like all great teachers, he embodied a bhakta's love. He addressed the 1893 Parliament of the World's Religions in Chicago several times, and you can access a powerful short recording of his opening remarks on Audible: "A Rare Recording of Swami Vivekananda." He founded the Vedanta Society in New York City the following year. There are now Vedanta Society centers in numerous U.S. cities. The monk serving as minister at the original Upper West Side location at the time of this writing is Swami Sarvapriyananda. He is so gifted with the ability to make complex concepts understandable, he has become a YouTube star on the Vedanta Society of New York channel.

Another noted jnani was author W. Somerset Maugham, whose semi-autobiographical novel and subsequent feature film, *The Razor's Edge*, is based on a passage from the Upanishads, those Indian scriptures that deal with philosophy and consciousness. If this path appeals, you may wish to read *Jnana Yoga*, by Swami Vivekananda, and *How to Practice Self Inquiry* or any of the other writings of Ramana Maharshi, an enlightened teacher of the last century.

One of these approaches may call to you and if it does, it may be all you need. Common this day and age is a comprehensive approach that accommodates all these. The yogi, or yogi-in-the-making, strives for calmness and connection through raja yoga, seeks to turn whatever work is before them into karma yoga, strives to love the Divine and all expressions of it (bhakti), and endeavors, in the spirit of jnana, to know who they are. This eclectic methodology may not be classic, but it suits contemporary, multi-tasking temperaments. In terms of aging like a yogi, all these paths and techniques are ways to focus on the present moment, an ageless state earmarked by all possibilities.

PRACTICES FOR THE PATH

Starting today, or this coming Monday if that makes more sense, spend one week doing all your work as a karma yogi would. Whether at your job, while volunteering, doing housework, or meeting family obligations, treat each task as if the Great Beneficence were your employer. And of course you would be right, whether or not karma yoga is your primary path.

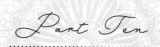

Part Ten

Warrior Challenges

Chapter 37

Dare to Live Fully

*Life is practice, practice is life. I commit to living my life
fully in this moment.*

....

JUDITH HANSON LASATER, AUTHOR OF *LIVING YOUR YOGA*

It is a rare asana class that doesn't include some variation of virabhadrasana, a warrior pose or series or flow. Some teachers translate virabhadrasana as "hero" instead of "warrior," but either way these postures exist to help us draw on inner strength, reserves of courage we may not remember that we possess. While life itself offers no shortage of challenges, we can choose to take on a warrior challenge by voluntarily stepping up to do something new, something different, something important. A warrior challenge may be daunting, but let's start with one that's fun: "Dare to live fully." Living fully is a keynote of youth and imparts youthfulness at any age. Besides, this is the youngest day of the rest of your life. Live it with gusto.

When I was forty-three, I went bungee jumping. It was thrilling. I entered into the experience with a fear of heights and afterwards felt like Superwoman. In addition, my daughter, Adair, a little girl at the time, was watching. She is now a professional aerialist and stunt performer, and I wonder if seeing her mom go through with that jump played some tiny part in the development of her own daring nature. In any case, two years later I injured my neck. There is quite a list of activities I haven't been able to do since, and bungee jumping is definitely on it. If I had waited, I would have missed that experience. Don't miss any that are earmarked for you.

A great way to start living fully is to look at people who are already doing it:

- Monica is one of the women in my building who is part of our twice-a-week yoga group. She lives an idyllic retired life with lots of travel, lots of family. Monica is Catholic, her husband is Hindu, and their children married a Muslim, a Jew, and a Protestant, so there is always a holiday to celebrate.

- Essie and Ann are a couple I admire. He is ninety-year-old physician Caldwell Esselstyn, Jr., MD, who wrote *Prevent and Reverse Heart Disease*, and Ann, a strength athlete at eighty-eight, coauthored with their daughter, Jane, *The Prevent and Reverse Heart Disease Cookbook*. The Esselstyns sometimes post photos and videos of themselves dancing. The joy in their connection, the movement, and the music is infectious.

- Suzanne Taylor entered my life via a pre-release copy of my book, *Shelter for the Spirit*. "This woman likes spiritual authors and she knows everybody," the publicist who sent her the book told me. "If she resonates with what you've written, she'll give you a party in LA." I believe we're now ten parties in. Suzanne was a successful actress in her twenties and thirties, but her passion was always to bring the world to a more enlightened place. More recently, then, she made a critically acclaimed documentary about crop circles, *What on Earth?* She puts on major speaker events and produces a plethora of imaginative projects to create community. I won't share her age, but you know mine and she has me beat.

- And Stella, of course, my lovely London yoga teacher who is close to 100, hosts a Sunday morning women's salon every week. The guest list is eclectic, and the only rule of the gathering is that no view is censored.

These people are young by every measure except chronology. You might also say that they are lucky to have good health and the genes for longevity. True. But this challenge is about maximum engagement in life, whatever your maximum is. If you have physical limitations or financial limitations, you have to work around those; just don't add on thought limitations.

I have another friend, Lane. Despite an unassailably healthful lifestyle, she became ill and is currently in assisted living. It took her a minute to adjust. Now, she engages maximally in life in her new situation. She is always telling me, "It's time for luncheon. I'll call you later," or "We are all going to the pub for drinks, but I'll find somewhere quiet to talk for a minute." (The pub, it seems, is onsite.) So much of this is attitude, an inner commitment to *carpe* some *diem* every chance you get. It may look as if it comes easy to some people, but life engagement takes effort for anyone who is no longer young. Those who live fully make the effort.

This might seem to stand in opposition to yogic teachings which imply that eschewing the world and meditating all day is a more efficient means to spiritual liberation. For some people, I'm sure it is. We are probably not those people. Yoga has always allowed two broad paths for seekers. One is to become a renunciate, spiritual by profession, and then there's everybody else, traditionally called "householders." That's us, regardless of the configuration of our household. We are the ones tasked with seeing the Divine in the midst of work and family, the noise and the news. We do this not by turning from the world but by seeing it as Holiness taking form. There's a lot out there that doesn't appear very holy, but the more we look for the Light, the lighter things get.

Our earthly experience, a mixed bag if there ever was one, is nevertheless more glorious than we are able to grasp while we're in it. There is an interactive Zen story which tells of a blind sea turtle who lives far out in a vast ocean. This creature comes to the surface of the water only once a century. We are then asked—this is the interactive part—to imagine that we are standing on the shore of that vast ocean fumbling about with a little wooden ring, an embroidery hoop, let's say, and just for the fun of it, we toss that small circle of wood out into the sea. The likelihood, the story goes, of that blind sea turtle's coming to the surface through our embroidery hoop is the likelihood of being given a human life.

When I think of that story, I am glad I went bungee jumping—and that I moved to England at eighteen and to New York at fifty. I am thrilled to pieces that I became a mom at thirty-three. I am grateful that I started a business in my sixties and am writing this book in my seventies. This kind of life engagement blocks attitudinal decrepitude. It grounds us in this moment where regrets about the past and fears about the future are not allowed. And it gives us memories: bright, vivid, colorful, entertaining, enchanting, enriching memories. If the time should come when the width of our life narrows significantly, its depth need not lessen at all.

PRACTICES FOR THE PATH

Let's end ageism. It is real and pervasive. As we grow older, we are almost certain to be subject to it, and for people who have already experienced racism, homophobia, or some other fear-borne bias, this adds an additional, oppressive layer. As with all prejudices, distrust of "the other" is at the root. Young folks, and some who aren't all that young, see the aged as a kind of under-caste.

Moreover, advancing age scares people. It is a reminder of the transience of this life. Some individuals––and some cultures, notably ours––find that diminishing older adults is easier than facing the reality that every human being is growing older every day. The message that needs to get out is this: *No matter how old we get, we will always be ourselves.* This means we'll always be whole, valid, and worthy of respect.

A first step is to diffuse the ageism within ourselves. We can, for instance, destigmatize objects that ought to be neutral: a cane, a walker, a hearing aid, an oxygen tank. These are simply tools that better the lives of a great many people, and they may do that for us one day. Can you start to see these as neutral, like a bicycle or a water bottle? Also, we can get to know people of advanced age, especially if we didn't have grandparents or great-grandparents in our lives as children. And we can steadfastly believe in ourselves and show up for ourselves as we mature: we'll be a lot less marginalized if we refuse to hang out at the margins. We can show up for others, too, those older than we are and those close to our age who are not able to enjoy the level of vitality and mobility that we presently do.

We can also show up politically. The arguments and deal-making around policy and regulation can seem antithetical to a yogic way of living, but Mahatma Gandhi used yoga's ethical principles to free his nation, and we can use them to lift the status of older people in our society. We need to move beyond tokenism in which we honor a few elders as national treasures and relegate everybody else to lessened status. It is our sacred trust to stand for full personhood for all, regardless of age (or any other descriptor for that matter). As yogis in progress, we are uniquely equipped to take the lead in this since we know that everybody is ageless anyway.

Chapter 38

Dare to Do Your Dharma

Everyone has been made for some particular work, and
the desire for that work has been put in every heart. Let
yourself be silently drawn by the stronger pull
of what you really love.

....

RUMI

Your *dharma* is your unique and personal work for this lifetime. It is essential for playing out your spiritual journey, and it is also how you contribute to the evolution of the universe. How stunning to ponder that with all our shortcomings and humanness, we have been tasked with something this monumental! You will sometimes hear the phrase "to co-create with God." This is how we do it.

Dharma translates as "duty," but it also implies destiny, your soul's assignment, your life's purpose. We can see these assignments easily in the lives of people who achieved something so impressive they're known around the world long after they leave it: *Harriet Tubman: Conduct the Underground Railroad . . . Orville and Wilbur Wright: Invent the airplane . . . Hedy Lamarr: Be a glamorous movie star and then come up with the technology that leads to Wi-Fi.*

But we are all more complex than even our greatest accomplishment, and our dharma shows this. It might include studying a particular subject, serving the world in a profession or business, raising a family, caring for elderly parents, effecting some social change, and seeking to know God. It is a lot, but we're not expected to tackle all of it at once—except for the knowing God part, aka, coming to know the Truth. This we work toward every day, no matter what else we're doing. As George Harrison said just before he died, "Everything else can wait, but the search for God cannot wait. And love one another."

Dharma is 100 percent customized. The fact that it is ours, more even than the fact that it is good, makes it our dharma. There are all kinds of good things to do and we can certainly assist in some of them. We can kick in a few bucks when a friend is doing a 10k run for their favorite charity. We can sign a petition for something important, even if it's not the most important thing to us. Your dharma, however, has your name on it. In the Bhagavad Gita (chapter 18, verse 47), Krishna tells Arjuna, "Better is one's own dharma, though imperfect, than the dharma of another well performed."

Reporting for our dharma is a warrior challenge because oftentimes doing anything else is more appealing. I sometimes think of dharma—what I'm here for—as akin to the priorities on my to-do list. The tasks that need to be taken care of first can be intimidating, so I am tempted to avoid them in favor of others: "Clear out some old pictures on your phone. Buy new yoga pants." There is nothing wrong with these but no self-respecting warrior would put them ahead of their dharma.

And never fall for the trap of "This is interesting. I wish I had known about it twenty years ago, but for me that ship has sailed." It has not sailed, because you are the ship. Your dharma is there for you to report for every day of your life. It doesn't matter if you didn't know the word early on; you knew what was expected and, for the most part, you did a darned good job of it, the very best you could. We all did. And now we know the word and the concept and its importance. With this further elucidation, we can report for duty today.

How you show up for your dharma will be different at different life stages. *That* you show up for it is required as long as you're breathing. "Take care of the baby" is a crucial dharmic command for anyone with a baby to care for, but when the children are grown and gone, there is another aspect of dharma to attend to. You can find yours today by simply asking God (or your Inner Teacher or Inner Light, whatever you call it) what your purpose is, both overall and at this specific time. If you're willing to be quiet and listen, the answer will be there for you. When you're in the flow of dharma, it just feels right, even if what you need to do calls for hard work and success is not guaranteed. Remember Joseph Campbell's "Follow your bliss"? It can be like that.

And it is a really big deal. Adi Shankara, the eighth century Vedic teacher and prolific writer, laid it out: "By fulfilling his dharma, a man marches along the path of progress until he attains the supreme dharma of all beings, namely, the realization of Truth." This is thrilling. It means that doing your job and making your art and being there for your family are spiritual practices, provided you allow them to be so through your attitude and dedication. This means your journey toward enlightenment is not confined to the time you spend on a yoga mat or meditation cushion. Great chunks of your daily life can contribute to the ultimate goal and enable you to bless others in the meantime.

PRACTICES FOR THE PATH

Set things to music. Chanting is a joyful part of yoga for many practitioners. Unlike meditation and other disciplines whose benefits accrue from daily practice, chanting bestows graces whenever performed, even if occasionally or for a short period of time. The uplift comes both when you yourself do the chanting, when you listen to others do it, or in the lovely hybrid, *kirtan*. This is devotional chanting most often accompanied by musical instruments and a responsive element that allows you to participate, as well as listen.

Chanting is often called japa, and that is correct, but japa is, more broadly, any repetition of a mantra that can be repeated either aloud or silently. The classic Sanskrit mantras were developed by sages who understood the power of sound to affect us physically, mentally, and spiritually. Holding a mantra soundlessly in meditation can be a profound experience, as well, and reams of research bear this out. Science has also confirmed that the focused state and rhythmic breathing brought about by audible chanting lowers blood pressure and boosts mood.

The simplest mantra to intone is the primordial sound, Om, sometimes spelled A-U-M to encourage enunciation of each component: ahh, ooo, mmm; it's often accompanied by shanti, peace. The chant *Hari Om* is believed to remove obstacles that can make life and growth more difficult. Another that resonates with me is "*Lokah samastah sukhino bhavantu*," calling for happiness and freedom for all living beings, and asking that the thoughts, words, and actions of our day contribute to universal peace and liberation.

YouTube is a treasure trove of chanting and kirtan. Among the better known kirtan singers in the West are Krishna Das and the late Alice Coltrane, whose husband was jazz legend John Coltrane. Another of my favorites is Dayashila Carrie Grossman. You know the phrase "voice of an angel"? Carrie has that.

The first time I heard yogic devotional chanting, I was seventeen. A big, open gathering was happening in a Kansas City park, and members of the International Society for Krishna Consciousness came with their drums and harmoniums, singing "*Hare Krishna. . .Hare Rama*" with great abandon. I joined in, all the while praying that I wasn't saying anything blasphemous. Of course I wasn't. All names of the Divine are names of the Divine. They are all holy. I have come to appreciate and benefit from the Sanskrit chants, yet I still resonate more naturally with Plácido Domingo singing Verdi's Requiem or The Edwin Hawkins Singers belting out "Oh Happy Day." That's allowed too.

Chapter 39

Dare to Make Peace with Mortality

Through knowing death we can hold a beacon of love for every moment that has just passed, for every friend who has lost a friend, for every child who has lost a parent. . . for any suffering anywhere.

....

SEBASTIAN POLE, AUTHOR OF

DISCOVERING THE TRUE YOU WITH AYURVEDA

Death is such a nuisance. It's hard to get here in the first place—ask any mother—and learning how to operate a body and cultivate a mind takes twenty years or more. We have little enough time as it is, and we spend a third of it in sleep. Even if we're blessed with longevity, indicators surface—cloudy vision, a bum knee, a senior moment—to remind us that we're only passing through.

Yoga is so insistent that we face the reality of death that *savasana,* the supine posture in which we restore ourselves and appropriate the benefits of asana class, means "corpse pose." This can seem morbid to Western sensibilities, so some books and teachers call it "sponge pose," but yoga contends that we need to practice for our death.

Meditation is another way to get some of this practice in. "Stoics and yogis both say that to overcome the fear of death one must think of it constantly in the proper manner," yoga practitioner David Presser writes in an article for YogaChicago.com. "Daily meditation involves withdrawing consciousness from the body—a preview of death." And as with anything else inevitable, we should prepare to exit with the most panache we can muster. This is the ultimate warrior challenge because it is the ultimate unknown, even though yoga says we're old hands at dying, having done it numerous times before.

Based on religious belief, scientific inquiry, or some intuitive glimmer, we all have different ideas about death and the afterlife. There is also a yogic view of death. Holding to it is not required—we said early on that yoga is far more a practice than a belief system. I personally resonate with the yogic view, as beautifully shared by yoga teacher and wellness consultant, Ashley Josephine Zuberi: "The cycle of the life of the soul is such that our spirit will continue to return until we transcend the cycle itself. This is enlightenment. Enlightenment can take many lifetimes... Ultimately the soul dissolves into everything, becomes omnipresent. It does not take physical form again. Instead, it permeates all beings."

It is intriguing to read about the deaths of realized individuals, jivanmuktas, people who came to full awareness of the truth of their being. These fully awakened ones live in the world as monks or mothers, dancers or doctors. When they pass, physical causes of death—illness, accident, or very advanced age—almost always exist, but these ordinary people who have become extraordinary participate in the process. They make a conscious exit: *mahasamadhi*—maha means "great."

We who are not yet enlightened and are likely to leave our bodies in more prosaic fashion can take heart in remembering that, like the realized being, we are not the body. Leaving aside philosophy and theology, our very cells are dying all the time. If we're talking only about the body, the child that we were, the teenager, the thirty-year-old are all dead. Except they're not. They are part of us. And I don't find it much of a stretch that we are part of all that is and that there is a point to everything, dying included.

"Death and dying," the academic discipline, is well named. Death is one thing, dying another. And for every individual, some amount of the resistance to the whole business can be apportioned to each category. As with so much else in life, preparation eases things. In a very practical way, every adult, even when young enough that dying is not supposed to happen, should have some exigency plans for healthcare, loved ones, and assets.

In terms of healthcare, a living will explains how you want to be treated in an emergency or if you otherwise cannot communicate your wishes. A durable power of attorney for healthcare makes someone you trust your health care proxy to communicate your desires to the hospital folks. Not everybody has both, but everybody needs one or the other. It's not fair to expect doctors and nurses to read minds. They're busy working miracles.

A will allocates wealth and possessions and can also spell out how any dependents (companion animals, for instance) will be cared for. Make it easier on the humans by having copies of necessary paperwork in a file or safe that the people close to you know about and can get into without a locksmith. They need easy access to your various passwords, as well. (There's a product call a Nokbox—short for "next of kin box"—that keeps all this stuff in order: www.nokbox.com.)

Even all prepped up, no one likes to think about sickness or pain, and we can take heart that hospice exists, making the dying process far more humane when death does not come quickly. There are even end-of-life doulas, or death doulas, trained to guide a dying person through the process the way a traditional doula guides a woman into motherhood. In addition, all religions have rituals and guidance for the end of life. Explore these, but don't become obsessed with death: If innumerable teachers are to be believed, it is merely passing through a door. Just don't avoid it either. Fear grows in darkness.

In chapter 8 of the Bhagavad Gita, Krishna tells Arjuna, and subsequently us, what to do when death is imminent. I recommend reading that chapter in its entirety. It is nothing less than a tutorial on how to proceed at the time of death, including in part: "With your mind completely stilled, free of selfish passions, and your concentration fixed at the third eye between your eyebrows, you will realize the supreme Lord. Close down the doors of the senses and place your mind in the heart. Then, while absorbed in meditation, focus all energy upward towards the head, repeating the sacred sound of Om, the sound of the eternal Godhead." I don't know about you, but I can face anything more easily when I have clear instructions.

> ### PRACTICES FOR THE PATH
>
> Do something this week to make peace with mortality. Google "living will" or read that eighth chapter of the Gita. Share memories of a deceased loved one with somebody who also loved them. Then plunge fully into this day, elated that you're here to live it.

Chapter 40

Dare to Elevate Everything

The world is a screen where we project our pictures. If we change and project love and peace, the world will change. People try to change the world without changing themselves. Only when we change will the world change.

....

DR. VASANT LAD, BAM&S, MASc

A great deal of yoga's value is in its uplift function. We see this as we perform postures—stand tall, stretch out, reach long—and in admonitions such as "Get *up* early. . .Clean *up* often. . .*Raise* your consciousness in meditation." The commitment to elevate everything uplifts our lives in the present moment, the way we'll meet our future, the lives of those around us, and, according to these sacred teachings, all life in the universe. It is, then, well worth the effort.

In the warrior challenge of elevating everything, you are called to keep your energy just a smidge higher than the energy around you. Each day offers opportunities to do this.

- You meet a friend for lunch who says, "I just don't see how the state of the world could get any worse." You might respond with, "The state of my world picked up the minute I saw you."
- You missed your bus and start to say, "Oh, sh-t!" but decide instead to be grateful that you get to sit—thirteen minutes of extra contemplation time, courtesy of your city's transportation department.

- You hear an ambulance siren and immediately you're in prayer mode, sending light and healing energy to a stranger who is, at his heart or her heart or their heart, the same divine expression as you are yourself.

Lately, during *yoga nidra*, deep relaxation at the end of an asana class, I find myself not in my living room with a laptop or at the Integral Yoga Institute in Greenwich Village, but at a second-floor studio in Manchester Street, London. I'm eighteen. When the teacher says, "Relax your feet," I hear the voice of Stella, my first yoga teacher. "Relax your calves. Relax your thighs." And it seems that the deeper I go, the younger I get.

I was telling the respected vaidya, Scott Gerson, MD, about this, and he said, "It sounds like a kind of *siddhi*." In Patanjali's Yoga Sutras, siddhis are supernatural powers yogis can develop. I don't give much thought to them because, although I aspire to be Self-realized one day, I'm not looking for otherworldly razzle-dazzle in the meantime. But I loved that Dr. Gerson said what he did, that even a yogic layperson like me, dogged by laziness and busyness and a mind prone to flit hither and yon, can create a little magic.

My rejuvenating, albeit imaginary, junkets to London as my body rests in New York are magical. You can call in magic too. Give somebody a little hope. Create a poem or a nonprofit or a pot of soup. Amaze your doctor by lowering your LDL with beans, rice, and sun salutations. Bend from your hips in full forward bend, reaching an eighth of a centimeter further than you did yesterday.

In your ability to elevate, you have a genuine opportunity to change the world. It's a great spiritual leap to embrace the reality that you cannot change another person or what took place in the past, but you can upgrade circumstances in this room at this moment. Smile and mean it. Make tea. Make conversation. Sweep up. Open a window. Play some music. Listen to someone. Scratch the cat's ears. Rub the dog's tummy. Want to change the world? You just did.

I find elevation far more effective than rules and chastisement for altering my behavior or, for that matter, anyone else's. Religions are known for "thou shalt not's," and yoga philosophy can carry the scourge of "Karma's gonna get you if you don't watch out." That is why I haven't spoken much about karma in this book, even though this vast teaching of justice and balance pervades the wisdom of the East. (It's not there exclusively, of course. St. Paul told the Galatians, "A man reaps what he sows.") So, yes, it's foolish to knowingly put forth anything harmful to another being—by action, word, or even thought.

On the other hand, we are still learning. You could chalk it up to karma, cause and effect, when a baby not yet adept at walking topples onto the rug. It is not punishment, just physics in action when a body is off balance. There's no blame or shame or gnashing of baby teeth. That's how I look at karma. I've done things I wish I hadn't, and while I can't claim the innocence of the teetering toddler, none of my regretful actions were taken with evil intent.

While I don't see it as some tit-for-tat point system, karma is part of my worldview. Without it, everything would seem random and point-less. We positively contribute to the world (i.e., elevate something) and a kind of energy is put forth that ultimately comes back to us in some way. If we act cruelly or selfishly, another energy goes out and some-how comes back, maybe in this life, maybe later. The good stuff we do can offset the not so hot and we are free to change our behavior, make restitution when called for, and reroute at least some portion of our des-tiny. I don't understand the precise workings of karma any more than I know who played the drum for the Big Bang, but it makes sense to live as well as we can. Besides, it feels better than being petty or selfish or mean-spirited.

Then there's grace. In the West, we think of this as forgiveness of sin, unmerited but bestowed with such depth of divine love, it wipes the slate clean. Yogic teachings in no way oppose grace—they imply that we live immersed in it—but in the yogic view, we are students, not sinners. "Life is a school," Dede told me time and again when I was growing up. In the Bhagavad Gita (4.37), Krishna gives a rather grace-filled expla-nation of karma when he says, "Just as the heat of fire burns all wood to ashes, the fire of knowledge burns all karma." And you know well by now that this knowledge is not information gathered and exams passed; it's the knowledge of our divine heritage and identity.

I suggest, then, that you make a mental note to elevate everything you can reach or touch or influence. After some time and focus on this, you'll do it merely by walking into a room. Your presence, like Iris's when we worked together in the Theosophical Society's library, can inspire someone so much that they'll write about it fifty years from now. And you will find yourself seeing beauty and grace and light in the most surprising places—today and when you're older than you thought you'd ever get. You will see beauty and grace and light in the serendipities of life, in your connections with other people, animals, and nature, and in your connection with the Divine. As far as I can tell from a lifetime of looking into this stuff, there is nothing better than that.

PRACTICES FOR THE PATH

Go forth into the rest of your life, determined to live by the words of this twentieth century Yogi:

- "When you come to a fork in the road, take it."
- "You can observe a lot just by watching."
- "Take it with a grin of salt."
- "It ain't over till it's over." —Yogi Berra

Brilliant Books

I must be disciplined about bibliographies or they could go on and on. I love books—reading them on paper, listening on audio, even just being around them in a bookstore or library. I stand behind every book mentioned or quoted within these pages, but I'm keeping myself in check here and listing only those that I continually read and use and love. I have put these in groups by subject matter, but several could fit in more than one category.

Aging

Asp, Karen, *Anti-Aging Hacks: 200+ Ways to Look and Feel Younger.* Adams Media, 2019.

Goddard, Jayney, *Rewind Your Body Clock: The Complete Natural Guide to a Happier, Healthier, Younger You.* Watkins, 2019.

Greger, Michael, MD, FACLM, *How Not to Age: The Scientific Approach to Getting Healthier as You Get Older.* Flatiron Books, 2023.

Leider, Richard J., and David A. Shapiro, *Who Do You Want to Be When You Grow Old? The Path to Purposeful Aging.* Berrett-Koehler Publishers, 2021.

Moran, Victoria, *Younger by the Day: 365 Ways to Rejuvenate Your Body and Revitalize Your Spirit.* HarperOne, 2004.

Asana and Pranayama

Le Page, Joseph, and Lillian Le Page, *Yoga Toolbox for Teachers and Students: Yoga Posture Cards for Harmonizing All Dimensions of Being.* Integrative Yoga Therapy, 2015.

Fishman, Loren, MD, *Healing Yoga: Proven Postures to Treat Twenty Common Ailments from Backache to Bone Loss, Shoulder Pain to Bunions, and More.* W.W. Norton, 2015. (See also Dr. Fishman's *Yoga for Arthritis, Yoga for Osteoporosis,* and *Yoga for Back Pain.*)

Satchidananda, Sri Swami, *The Breath of Life: Integral Yoga Pranayama.* Integral Yoga Publications, 2015.

Sivananda Yoga Vedanta Centre, *Yoga Mind and Body.* DK Publishing, 2008.

Stiles, Tara, *Yoga Cures: Simple Routines to Conquer More Than 50 Common Ailments and Live Pain-Free.* Harmony Books, 2012.

Ayurveda

Chopra, Deepak, MD, *Perfect Health: The Complete Mind Body Guide.* Three Rivers Press, 2000.

Frawley, David, MD, *Yoga and Ayurveda: Self-Healing and Self-Realization.* Lotus Press, 2009.

Kucera, Sarah, DC, CAP, *The Ayurvedic Self-Care Handbook: Holistic Healing Rituals for Every Day and Season.* The Experiment, 2019.

Raichur, Pratima, and Mariam Cohn, *Absolute Beauty: Radiant Skin and Inner Harmony Through the Ancient Secrets of Ayurveda.* William Morrow Paperbacks, 1999.

Sivananda Yoga Vedanta Center, *Practical Ayurveda: Find Out Who You Are and What You Need to Bring Balance to Your Life.* DK Publishing, 2018.

Snyder, Kimberly, and Deepak Chopra, MD, *Radical Beauty: How to Transform Yourself from the Inside Out.* Harmony Books, 2016.

Biographies (or biographically enhanced nonfiction)

Corn, Seane, *Revolution of the Soul: Awaken to Love Through Raw Truth, Radical Healing, and Conscious Action.* Sounds True, 2019.

Goldberg, Michelle, *The Goddess Pose: The Audacious Life of Indra Devi, the Woman Who Helped Bring Yoga to the West.* Knopf, 2015.

Puerta, Tatiana Forero, *Yoga for the Wounded Heart: A Journey, Philosophy, and Practice of Healing Emotional Pain.* Lantern Books, 2018.

Saraswati, Sadhvi Bhagawati, *Hollywood to the Himalayas: A Journey of Healing and Transformation*. Mandala Publishing, 2021.

Swami, Radhanath, *The Journey Home: Autobiography of an American Swami—Mystics, Yogis, Gurus, and an Epic Quest Through Spiritual India*. Mandala Publishing, 2010.

Yogananada, Paramahansa, *Autobiography of a Yogi*. Self-Realization Fellowship, 12th ed., 1994.

Cookbooks

Dodge, Tamal, and Victoria Dodge, *The Yoga Plate: Bring Your Practice into the Kitchen with 108 Simple & Nourishing Vegan Recipes*. Sounds True, 2019.

Gannon, Sharon, *Simple Recipes for Joy: More Than 200 Delicious Vegan Recipes*. Avery, 2014.

Ketabi, Sahara Rose, *Eat Feel Fresh: A Contemporary Plant-Based Cookbook*. DK Publishing, 2018.

Lutzker, Talya, *The Ayurvedic Vegan Kitchen: Finding Harmony Through Food*. Book Publishing Company, 2012.

Plant-based Lifestyle

Adams, Carol J., Patti Breitman, and Virginia Messina, MPH, RD, *Never Too Late to Go Vegan: The Over-50 Guide to Adopting and Thriving on a Plant-Based Diet*. The Experiment, 2014.

Gannon, Sharon, *Yoga and Veganism: The Diet of Enlightenment*. Mandala Publishing, 2020.

Greger, Michael, MD, FACLM, with Gene Stone, *How Not to Die: Discover the Foods Scientifically Proven to Prevent and Reverse Disease*. Flatiron Books, 2015.

McQuirter, Tracye, and Mary McQuirter, *Ageless Vegan: The Secret to Living a Long and Healthy Plant-Based Life*. DaCapo Lifelong Books, 2018.

Reinfeld, Mark, and Ashley Boudet, ND, *The Ultimate Age-Defying Plan: The Plant-Based Way to Stay Mentally Sharp and Physically Fit*. DaCapo Press, 2019.

Satchidananda, Sri Swami, *The Yoga Way: Food for Body, Mind and Spirit*, rev. by Carole Baral et al. Integral Yoga Publications, 2017.

Turner, Paul Rodney, *Food Yoga: Nourishment for Body, Mind, & Soul*, rev. ed. Food Yoga International, 2013

Yoga Philosophy

Adele, Deborah, *The Yamas and Niyamas: Exploring Yoga's Ethical Practice*. On-Word Bound Books, LLC, 2009.

Easwaran, Eknath, *The Bhagavad Gita*. Nilgiri Press, 2009. (See also Easwaran's translation of *The Upanishads* and *The Dhammapada*, and his *Original Goodness: A Commentary on the Beatitudes*.)

Lasater, Judith, PhD, P.T. *Living Your Yoga: Finding the Spiritual in Everyday Life*. Rodmell Press, 2000.

Prabhavananda, Swami, and Christopher Isherwood, *How to Know God: The Yoga Aphorisms of Patanjali*. Vedanta Press, 2007.

Viljoen, Edward, *The Bhagavad Gita: The Song of God Retold in Simplified English*. St. Martin's Essentials, 2019.

Acknowledgments and Permissions

This book would not exist but for the belief and tenacity of my agent, Matthew Carnicelli, and my editor, Jon Sweeney. I'm so happy the two of you hit it off so *Age Like a Yogi* could find the perfect home at Monkfish Books. Thanks to you both, and to legendary spiritual books publisher Paul Cohen and gifted and generous designer, Colin Rolfe, for his design of both the cover and the interior of this book.

I owe tremendous gratitude to Sharon Gannon, whom I admire to the moon and back, for contributing her thoughtful foreword, and to everyone who provided a personal epigraph or a testimonial. Others who helped make *Age Like a Yogi* happen include Heather Dahman, Camille DeAngelis, Marty Davey, MS, RD, Susan Deninger, Marie Doré, Dominique Guerin, Elaine Hutchison, Cristen Iris, Jessica Krant, MD, Sarah Kucera, DC, CAP, Helene Lynn, Sande Nosonowitz, Holly Skodis, Jim Spellos, and Cindy Thompson, plus ongoing support from the Tuesday/Thursday morning yoga core group: Monica Baliga, Verrie Grey, Annelee Ochel, and Suhrita Sen.

In addition, I want to thank the coterie of authors who agreed to proofread a chapter or two or several: Nathaniel Altman, Karen Asp, Rev. Sarah Bowen, Patti Breitman, Joann Farb, Leslie Levine, Martin Rowe, Rev. Carol Saunders, Deborah Shouse, and Ruby Warrington.

Appreciation also goes to everyone at Tantor Audio for the production of the audio version of this book, and to Marybeth Lynch, CCC-SLP, and Eunice Wong for helpful tutelage on reading the book for the recording.

I am incredibly grateful to my recent teachers, who planted within me the concepts that would become *Age Like a Yogi*: Richard Masla of the Ayurveda Health Retreat, Alachua, Florida, my first formal teacher of ayurveda; Syama Masla, Jai Giridhari, Dhyana Masla, and Vira Tansey of the Bhakti Center, New York City, who conducted the yoga teacher training I took at 70; and Swami Karunananda of Integral Yoga (Yogaville, Virginia), head teacher of the raja yoga teacher training I was part of the following year. There is much of all of you in these pages.

If I named everyone I consider a spiritual guide who brought me to the point of writing *Age Like a Yogi*, it would take another book-length work, but my life is full of teachers. If I know you and you're noted or quoted elsewhere in this book, I haven't repeated your name here to save space, but please know that I appreciate you deeply. And although I know I'm leaving people out—it's a lapse of memory, not a lapse of love—some mentors and guides not otherwise named include Alison Adler, Linda Adler, Sherry Boone, Rachel Borkowski, Kris Carlson, Judy Carman, Fran Costigan, Elizabeth Cutting, Philippe DeJean, Freya Dinshah, Beth Ertz, Linda Flake, Necia Gamby, Carlos Garcia, Marian Hailey-Moss, Rosalind Graham, Suzanne Hatlestad, Jacinta Jayadevi Hollon, Richard Horwege, Lydia Huston, Kevin Kelly, Guruparwaz Khalsa, Stan Krajewski, Judy Kretmar, Joy Lawrence, Durga Leela, Danielle Legg, Lisa Levinson, Linda Long, Rev. Chris Michaels, Panchali Null, John Pierre, Joy Pierson, Mary Rouse, Rita Rousseau, Jiten Ruparel, PhD, Dolores Sehorn, Carol Shiflett, Louann Stahl, Suzanne Tague, Rev. Paul Tenaglia, Rev. Duke Tufty, Stephanie Sri Wegman, Jacqueline Whitmore, and Kimberly Wilson.

There are others who have passed away: Valda Anderson, Carole Baral, Richard Carlson, PhD, Adelene DeSoto, Donna Hart, Donna Henes, Frankie Grady, Gladys Lawler, Gladys Marshall, James Melton, Dr. Patrick Moran, Robert Morris, Jerrold Mundis, Lucia Robinson, and Iris White.

Thanks to my daughter and son-in-law, Adair and Nick Moran (yes, he took her name), for inspiring me with their incredible commitment to living fully, working hard, and going for impossible dreams until they become possible. And to Nick's parents, Drs. George and Carol Little: bless you for inviting me to your inviting home for the writer's retreat that meant I was able to turn in the manuscript on time. Thanks to William's children, Siân Melton and Erik Melton, for welcoming in an eccentric stepmom over twenty-five years ago and giving me the great gift of more family. And finally, immense gratitude goes to my husband, Rev. William Melton for your own spiritual awakening, your inspiring grasp of ahimsa, and your unwavering belief in this book, its message, and its writer. I know it is not easy to live with an author on deadline, and you have done it eleven times now.

***

Indian chocolate shake recipe reprinted with permission, with acknowledgment to *The Ayurvedic Vegan Kitchen: Finding Harmony Through Food* by Talya Lutzger, published by the Book Publishing Company, P.O. Box 69, Summertown, TN, USA 38483. ©2012. All rights reserved.

Ayurvedic facial care routine reprinted with permission, with acknowledgment to *Ayurvedic Beauty Care: Ageless Techniques to Evoke Natural Beauty* by Melanie A. Sachs, published by Lotus Press, P.O. Box 325, Twin Lakes, WI, USA 53181. ©1994. All rights reserved.

....

Victoria Moran is a longtime devotee of yoga and author of 13 previous books on wellbeing, compassionate living, and eclectic spirituality.
Creating a Charmed Life was an international bestseller, and *Shelter for
the Spirit* and *Lit from Within* earned her spots on The Oprah Winfrey
Show. Victoria hosts the *Main Street Vegan Podcast*, is founder and direc-
tor of Main Street Vegan Academy, and a cofounder of the Compassion
Consortium, an interfaith spiritual center based on the principle of
ahimsa. She was, at age 66, voted Peta's Sexiest Vegan Over 50, and
in her early 70s trained as a yoga instructor (RYT-200) and raja yoga
instructor. Victoria is a frequent speaker and podcast guest, based in
New York City.